SNAKE OIL IS ALIVE AND WELL

THE CLASH BETWEEN MYTHS AND REALITY: REFLECTIONS OF A PHYSICIAN

by

MORTON E. TAVEL, MD

Published by
Brighton Publishing LLC
501 W. Ray Road
Suite 4
Chandler, Arizona 85225

SNAKE OIL IS ALIVE AND WELL
The Clash between Myths and Reality:
Reflections of a Physician

by

Morton E. Tavel, MD

Clinical Professor of Medicine
Indiana University School of Medicine
Consulting Cardiologist, St. Vincent Hospital
Indianapolis, IN

Published by

Brighton Publishing LLC
501 W. Ray Road
Suite 4
Chandler, Arizona 85225

First Edition

Printed in the United States of America

Copyright 2012

ISBN 13: 978-1-936587-88-9

ISBN 10: 1-936-58788-2

Cover Design by Tom Rodriguez

All rights reserved. No part of this publication may be reproduced or transmitted in any form or by any means, electronic or mechanical, including photocopy, recording, or any information storage retrieval system, without permission in writing from the copyright owner.

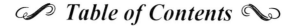 *Table of Contents*

ᑳᔈ *Acknowledgements* ᥅ᣞ

The author wishes to express his gratitude to the following individuals for valuable assistance and support in the creation and preparation of this manuscript:

Hart Katz, MD, PhD, President, SigmaTelemed, Inc.

Roy Amiet, PhD, cited for excellence in aeroacoustical engineering (AIAA)

Robert Hurwitz, MD, Clinical Professor of Medicine, Indiana University School of Medicine

Kenneth Oldfield, MA, PhD, Professor of Public Administration, University of Illinois-Springfield

Harriet Hall, MD, science writer and contributing editor to Skeptic and Skeptical Inquirer publications. Editor of website, Science Based Medicine.

Stephen Barrett, M.D. author, editor of website, Quackwatch, and consumer advocate, vice-president of the Institute for Science in Medicine and a Fellow of the Committee for Skeptical Inquiry.

"The fact that an opinion has been widely held is no evidence whatever that it is not utterly absurd; indeed in view of the silliness of the majority of mankind, a widespread belief is more likely to be foolish than sensible."

Bertrand Russell

◯ *Foreword* ◯

"I do not feel obliged to believe that the same god who has endowed us with sense, reason and intellect has intended us to forgo their use."

Galileo Galilei

Astronomer and Physicist, 1564—1642

If one stands in a forest filled with pseudoscientific beliefs, non sequiturs, major biases, and fundamentalist religious beliefs, is there anyone out there who will listen to explanations of valid science—especially science involving health issues? Whoever tries to impart such information may achieve an outcome as ill-fated as that of Don Quixote; but if there are at least a few listeners out there, my efforts will not have been in vain.

First we must explain the ingredient in this book's title, snake oil, which originated as a purported remedy in ancient China as a touted cure for arthritis. Chinese laborers on the gangs building the first Transcontinental Railroad gave snake oil to their coworkers, stating that when rubbed over painful joints, it would provide relief. Their claim was derided by rival medicine salesmen, and soon became a generic term for all types of quackery, in particular any product with exaggerated marketing hype but questionable or absent benefit. The snake-oil peddler later became a stock character in Western films—a traveling "doctor" with dubious credentials, selling snake oil (or a similar fake remedy) as a general panacea. The sales pitch was accompanied by boisterous marketing hype, which was often supported by pseudo-scientific evidence. To provoke enthusiasm and increase sales, an accomplice (shill) in the crowd would vouch for the product by citing his or her own miraculous cure. After bilking as many customers as possible, the doctor would prudently leave town before his customers realized that they'd been cheated.

One need not look far to see that the snake oil concept endures to this day, assuming such guises as alternative medicine, faith healing, fraudulent medical claims in the media, and information touted by "medical gurus" who can provide no scientific substantiation for their claims. Today's versions of snake oil, however, differ from the old stereotype in one important way; most individuals buying these products truly believe they are effective, meaning the peddler need not leave town in a hurry. This gullibility is not only widespread, but also seems to be gaining more traction, at least in the United States.

Consider the robust growth of alternative medicine. According to a 2007 survey of adults and children conducted by the CDC's (Centers for Disease Control and Prevention) National Center for Health Statistics (NCHS) and the National Center for Complementary and Alternative Medicine (NCCAM), 74.6% of the US population has used some form of alternative remedy in the past, and almost four out of ten had done so within the preceding twelve months.

How do we explain this lack of sophistication among a large segment of our populace? To answer this question, we must first delve into several underlying principles of human thought, among which are how judgments are formed that cause us to adopt biases; how we derive conclusions—true or false—from simple numerical and statistical concepts; how one determines causes when confronted by apparent effects; and what is really meant by the scientific concepts *hypothesis*, *theory*, and *proof*. We will address these and other issues later.

As a medical practitioner, I am disturbed by the volume of misinformation—especially about health matters—that now exist in all forms of communication. It is unwittingly provided by those who lack the tools to differentiate between truth and falsehood, and deliberately by self-serving individuals who should know better. We, as a society, are regularly subjected to all sorts of sound bites regarding so-called major breakthroughs about useless or unproven treatments. These are furnished to the public by purveyors of alternative methods, among other hoaxes, unsubstantiated by standard scientific criteria. These are modern-day reincarnations of snake oil.

In this book, I attempt to explain why we are so often willing to slavishly follow the spurious advice of experts—especially in matters of health—despite the fact that we have no concrete knowledge of their credentials, nor understand how their conclusions are drawn.

These fallacies of thought extend far beyond issues of health as related to encounters between caregivers and patients. Inspired by the abundance of misconceptions around me, I have focused this analysis on both the general public and the medical community. I present an overview of the evolution of medical science over the past two-hundred years, how the underlying thought patterns in health care have changed to overcome biases and superstitions, culminating in rigorous critical scientific thought patterns, and finally arriving at our present destination, *evidence-based medicine* (EBM) or *evidence-based practice* (EBP). Although rather messy at times, medical science has made the arduous and lengthy transition from superstition, myth, and doubtful logic to a discipline firmly grounded in scientific principles. Patterns of thought derived from this journey can be useful to the population at large, and can even extend to a better understanding of sporting events, the gambling casino, the financial markets, and even to political and world affairs.

Valid information about health and scientific matters is readily available almost everywhere—the internet, periodicals, and books, to name but a few. Books written by so-called medical experts provide us with factoids about such health issues as proper diets, exercise, health-promoting lifestyles, vitamins, drugs and their side effects, but many of their conclusions are not supported by evidence. Unfortunately, many people lack the necessary skills to help them separate the wheat from the chaff, because they lack the critical faculties and skepticism to question the claims and understand how to arrive at rational conclusions. Through modern physical and psychological science, we can identify the sources of many biases and myths and understand why they persist. These same principles can also help prevent the individual from falling prey to potentially deleterious health, social, financial, and other unfavorable outcomes.

At the crux of these issues is the need to understand the process of science and the need for skeptical thinking. As Carl Sagan, renowned astronomer and astrophysicist wrote in his book *The Demon-Haunted World*, "Skepticism does not sell well. A bright and curious person who relies entirely on popular culture to be informed about something like Atlantis is hundreds or thousands of times more likely to come upon a fable treated uncritically than a sober and balanced assessment." Sagan also notes that surveys find that some 95% of Americans are "scientifically illiterate." I believe that the average individual who pays lip service to the wonders of science has little interest in and less understanding of scientific methodology.

Members of the scientific community must be skeptics by nature. Their realm is limited to observable phenomena, and they regularly generate hypotheses and test them experimentally. After experimentation, they must then evaluate and criticize their own conclusions, consider alternative explanations, and defend their findings before their peers. Members of this latter group must question their results and attempt to provide alternative explanations and often construct other experiments to confirm or refute the initial findings. Conversely, the general public, wishing to obtain simple and direct answers to complex questions in the least time possible time, usually has little interest in the scientific method. Thus there is little general interest in—and even less understanding of—protracted discussions by scientists, who seem indecisive or overly circumspect. Christopher Toumey, in *Conjuring Science,* summarizes this problem by saying, "Good science makes bad television." Sadly, the converse is also true; bad science makes good television.

So, what are the advantages of learning to be skeptical? There are several, especially when it comes to matters of health:

1. The mental challenge associated with an incredulous approach can be stimulating and rewarding.

2. A better understanding of medical science leads to the proper analysis, interpretation, and rejection of the reports put forth by purveyors of misinformation, including, to a certain degree, major pharmaceutical companies.

3. Critical analysis and rejection of myths surrounding indeterminate phenomena such as extrasensory perception, communication with the dead, and extraterrestrials, will lead to a more secure—and less scary—existence.

4. Skepticism can prevent the waste of much hard-earned money, which should result in avoidance of countless useless remedies, unnecessary vitamins and supplements, and expensive designer drugs promoted heavily in the media by the pharmaceutical industry.

The purpose of this book, therefore, is to clarify the philosophy of science. This involves the acquisition of objective and measurable information, then subjecting it to rigorous analysis and debate. This is analogous to Galileo's use of evidence to support and establish the fact that the earth is not center of the solar system/universe. Although his theory got him into serious trouble with the church, in the long run his evidence carried the day (and night).

Although I provide many facts resulting from scientific inquiry, my objective is to explain the methods behind this science, thereby allowing the reader to be better able to identify what is valid and to reject what is not. In the process, I wish to provide a healthy dose of skepticism in a sea of uncritical thought, which will, hopefully, provide some counterbalance.

I dedicate this volume to all skeptics, and hope to recruit many new ones.

SECTION ONE: GENERAL BIASES AND PITFALLS

⸎ *Chapter One* ⸎

THE STRUGGLE BETWEEN SCIENCE AND "LOGIC": AN EXAMPLE

"Perfect as the wing of a bird may be, it will never enable the bird to fly if unsupported by the air. Facts are the air of science. Without them a man of science can never rise."

Ivan Pavlov

On a crisp, cool evening in late November, Brad Summers, fifty-two years of age, was about to experience a medical emergency that would nearly cost him his life. But as the story unfolds, an intriguing question arises: How much would his medical care have been compromised if it had been based upon myths rather than sound scientific underpinnings?

Brad had always enjoyed reasonably good health, but in recent years he'd gained about thirty pounds. At the same time, he'd noticed a bit of middle-age spread. Until he was about thirty-years-old, he'd exercised regularly by playing tennis and swimming. Before that, he'd played football in high school, playing the quarterback position with decent success.

Also during his high-school days, prompted by his contemporaries—and because it seemed "cool"—he'd started smoking cigarettes. He continued to smoke despite the objections of his wife, Jenny, and their two sons, rationalizing that—despite the package warning labels—a few of his friends were also still smoking and seemingly enjoying good health. Besides, the allegedly bad consequences mostly affected other people, and if a serious need arose, he could give it up.

After he turned forty, he became increasingly involved in business affairs, which led to him becoming almost totally sedentary. His diet was inconsistent, for his tight schedule frequently allowed only a visit to a fast-food restaurant to grab a burger. To compensate for his dietary shortcomings, he took multi-vitamin tablets.

His personal physician, whom he'd been seeing periodically, found him in reasonably good health, except for mild elevations in blood pressure and cholesterol. In addition to urging him to stop smoking, his doctor prescribed a drug to control his blood pressure and suggested that he go on a modified calorie-restricted diet to reduce his weight and cholesterol level. Since he felt well, Brad had trouble remembering to take the blood pressure medication, often missing single or multiple days. He found dieting was extremely difficult and did not lose weight. He also felt powerless over his smoking habit.

That fateful night in November, Brad was attending a high-school basketball game in which one of his sons was playing. The game was close, and everyone was cheering wildly, but during the last five minutes of the game, Brad's emergency began. He suddenly felt heavy pressure in the middle of his chest and upper abdomen, became nauseated, and began to perspire profusely. His wife, noting this apparent distress, asked him what was wrong. He said he "must have indigestion." Within seconds, however, he slumped over, gasped two or three times, and lost consciousness. His wife began to scream, after which a hush came over the gymnasium.

A nearby spectator, recognizing what had happened, quickly came to Brad's aid. Noting his unresponsiveness and the absence of a pulse, he quickly moved Brad onto the hard, flat surface of the floor and began cardiopulmonary resuscitation (CPR), applying rhythmic pressure with both palms over the middle of Brad's chest and administering mouth-to-mouth ventilation$^{\pm}$. At the same time, he instructed another spectator to call 911.

In less than five minutes, they heard sirens blaring as an ambulance approached, followed shortly by the entrance of two paramedical personnel armed with life-support equipment. Within seconds, they confirmed that Brad's heartbeat had assumed a chaotically irregular rhythm called *ventricular fibrillation*. They immediately placed two flat paddles connected to an *automated external defibrillator* (AED) on his chest, and administered an electrical shock which caused Brad's entire body to jerk. Checking again, the medics determined that Brad's heart had begun to contract rhythmically again, and his pulse had returned. But he had fallen unconscious because of the temporary cessation of blood flow to his brain. When effective heart action was restored, he began to mumble and make purposeful body motions, suggesting that irreversible brain damage may have been avoided. Only additional time, however, could provide information about how much mental function would return.

The ambulance then transported Brad to the nearest large metropolitan hospital, whereupon he was quickly evaluated in the emergency department (ED), also commonly called the emergency room (ER). An *electrocardiogram* (ECG) taken in this area showed that he had sustained a *myocardial infarction* (MI), or "heart attack.," which is the process of sudden damage to the heart resulting from cessation of blood flow from an obstructed artery responsible for supplying blood to this organ. Having already been alerted of his imminent arrival, the specially trained personnel of the cardiac division prepared the *cardiac catheterization* laboratory for the next phase of Brad's treatment. He was then taken promptly to this laboratory for further management.

$^{\pm}$ In instances of cardiac arrest, the need for mouth-to-mouth ventilation is controversial, believed by some authorities to be an unnecessary component of CPR.

By this time, Brad had regained consciousness and was still having chest discomfort, although it was less intense. He was moved to an uncomfortably hard, narrow table for a *cardiac catheterization*. During this procedure, a cardiologist placed a thin tube, or *catheter*, into the large artery in his groin and threaded it, quickly and painlessly, under x-ray guidance, to his heart and into the openings of his *coronary arteries*, which supply blood to the heart muscle. Next, a liquid material, or dye, was injected selectively into these arteries to obtain moving images of the interiors of the vessels via x-ray. These pictures demonstrated that one of the main coronary arteries supplying blood to the front of his heart was totally blocked by a blood clot, which cut off the blood supply to part of the heart muscle. Additionally, portions of this artery and the artery supplying other regions of his heart also showed areas of irregular partial narrowing, but they did not seem to be causing significant reduction of blood flow.

Less than an hour had transpired since the onset of Brad's chest pain, and this favorably short time lapse meant that, if the blockage could be relieved by restoration of blood flow to the jeopardized area of heart muscle, damage to the heart could be minimized or even prevented entirely. To do this, a special catheter with an inflatable balloon tip was placed into the blocked artery and inflated (angioplasty). The obstructed area opened readily and, after this was confirmed by x-ray, a *stent*, or small, firm sleeve, was placed at the site of this previous blockage to insure the vessel would remain unobstructed.

As soon as the vessel was opened, Brad noted the almost magical disappearance of his chest pain. After receiving additional medications to prevent further clotting and to slow the heart in order to reduce its metabolic needs, he was transferred to a special holding area (*coronary care unit*) containing cardiac monitoring equipment, and for the next five days he was observed and cared for by specialized personnel, who watched virtually every heartbeat for evidence of irregularity or other change. In two days, he was allowed to sit in a chair, and shortly thereafter he began to walk and engage in light exercise with supervision.

By his second day in the hospital, after having been groggy, Brad's mind had cleared completely, but he had little recollection for what had occurred at the time of his emergency. Because of this, he was eager to learn what had happened. His cardiologist, Dr. Ernest Thatcher, who had removed the obstruction in his coronary artery, explained in detail the events leading to his current situation. After hearing this, Brad had many questions.

"Why did a blood clot form in my heart in the first place?"

"The clot formed in a roughened area caused by a plaque of fatty material in the vessel wall. For reasons we don't entirely understand, the plaque's contents broke through a thin outer covering, which allowed them to interact with the blood, producing a clot that obstructed the blood flow."

"But you said there were plaques in other areas of my coronary arteries. Am I at risk for a repeat of this?"

"Yes, you are, but now that we're aware of this problem, we're giving you medication to reduce the chances of that happening. We've also started you on a drug to reduce your cholesterol. Studies indicate that this will also reduce the chances of a repeat episode. When combined with changes in your diet, cessation of smoking, and good control of your blood pressure, those plaques, which are found in most people's arteries, will begin to shrink and be less likely to cause trouble in the long run. This will affect obstructions not only in your heart, but also in your brain, kidneys and extremities."

Brad, thinking his case was unique, then asked, "How often does this sudden stoppage of heart activity occur?"

The doctor quickly launched into a monologue. "All too often. In the United States alone, this event occurs nearly a thousand times a day. Unfortunately, the vast majority of those who suffer such an episode do not survive, unless they occur in places where lots of people are present. Sometimes death can be averted by the use of *automated external defibrillators*, or 'AEDs', which are usually present in congested areas of airports, stadiums, and the like. You were very lucky indeed, because someone knew CPR and was able to keep blood moving to all your vital organs. That bought time until you could be 'defibrillated', which wiped clean the chaotic impulses running through your heart. That allowed your heart to resume a normal and effective rhythm. If AEDs are available, they're easy to use, even in the absence of trained medical personnel. They contain software that automatically determines the heart's activity and the need to apply the electrical shock."

The doctor added, "The same thing undoubtedly caused the untimely and sudden death of Tim Russert, newsman and NBC News's Washington bureau chief. He died suddenly at work, possibly because emergency aid wasn't quickly available."

Then came a critical question; Brad asked, "When, if ever, can I return to full physical activity?"

"I'm glad you asked," replied the doctor. "Contrary to what you may be thinking, you'll be put in a cardiac rehabilitation program and gradually increase your physical fitness to the point that, within several weeks, you'll be better conditioned than you've been in twenty years. You'll also learn about lifestyle changes that include proper diet, smoking cessation and others. Evidence shows that people who adhere to these changes actually enjoy a substantial lowering of long-term mortality," replied the doctor.

Brad sighed in obvious relief, but still had one more question. "Did emotional tension play any role in my attack, from either the excitement of the game or the long-term stress of my job?"

After a brief pause and a mildly perplexed look, the doctor replied, "That's a difficult question to answer. Although cardiac mortality temporarily rises in populations during periods of stress, such as natural disasters, and is more apt to occur in people who have high-pressure occupations, the real culprit here is *arteriosclerosis,* or hardening of the arteries. This is a process of irregular deposition of plaque-like material on the inner linings of the arteries, sometimes chronically restricting the flow of blood, commonly to the heart muscle. Stress may act as a trigger to acute events such as chaotic heart rhythm or the formation of blood clots, but we don't clearly understand the underlying dynamics in many of the cases. Also, stress itself is individually determined and virtually impossible to quantify. What seem to be severe external pressures may not be particularly stressful to some individuals. On the other hand, minor environmental disruptions may cause other predisposed persons to have exaggerated, even near-panic, internal reactions. Since we know that chronic internalized anxiety, hostility, and depression are markers of a greater risk for a poor long-term outcome, active treatment, including medication and psychiatric support, can improve emotional status and relieve symptoms. Unfortunately, there's no convincing evidence that treating or avoiding external stress can avert bad outcomes."

Having been convinced he had a new lease on life, Brad resolved to adhere closely to the program laid out before him, including all the recommended lifestyle changes. He only regretted that he'd not made such changes earlier so he could have avoided his present situation.

Brad was discharged from the hospital eight days later, with the medications to prevent further clotting, reduce the heart's energy requirements, and reduce his blood cholesterol. Two weeks later, he entered a supervised exercise program at the hospital, which he attended for one hour three times a week, during which his heart rate and rhythm were carefully monitored. He also received detailed counseling about diet and lifestyle changes.

One year later, he'd lost thirty pounds, his blood pressure and cholesterol were normal, and he'd continued to exercise regularly. He'd also been able to stop smoking, although not without difficulty. Follow-up tests showed that his heart function had returned to normal, with no evidence of residual damage. He did indeed feel better than he had in twenty years.

HOW MEDICAL SCIENCE REACHED THIS POINT

In early days of the twentieth century, individuals suffering from Brad's symptoms—chest pains radiating upward from the abdomen, accompanied by nausea—were often diagnosed as having "acute indigestion," or gallbladder or other intestinal problems, which seemed "logical". But medical practitioners of the day were at a loss to explain why many such persons died—often suddenly—from what was, apparently, a digestive disorder.

In 1912, however, an astute researcher named James B Herrick[1] observed, on post-mortem examinations, that blood clots were regularly present in one or more coronary arteries of individuals who died after experiencing such symptoms. He also recognized the need for a reliable diagnostic test to uncover the underlying condition. That test was the recently discovered electrocardiogram (ECG). This test remains the primary means of diagnosis today.

THE FRAMINGHAM HEART STUDY

During the first half of the 20th century, population studies showed that cardiovascular disease was rapidly ascending to its current position as the leading cause of death in the U.S., but little was known about why it was happening. All this began to change after 1948, when an ambitious research project was started in the small Massachusetts community of Framingham. In 1971, this

---

[1] Herrick JB. *Clinical features of sudden obstruction of the coronary arteries.* J. Am. Med. Assoc. 1912.59:2015-2020. Reprinted as a Landmark Article, Vol. 250, Oct 7, 1983.

study became a joint collaboration between the National Heart, Lung, and Blood Institute (NHLBI) and Boston University. Its objective was to identify common features that contribute to cardiovascular disease by following its development over a long period in a large group of participants who had not yet developed any evidence of this disease or had a previous heart attack or stroke. The researchers recruited 5,209 men and women between the ages of thirty and sixty-two, and began extensive physical examinations and lifestyle interviews that they later analyzed for common patterns related to disease development. Since then, surviving subjects have returned to the study every two years for a detailed medical examination and laboratory tests. In 1971, a second generation was enrolled—5,124 of the original participants' adult children and their spouses—to participate in the study. Since 1994, it has been expanded to include third-generation members of the same community, as well as groups with more varied genetic and racial backgrounds.

Over the years, information from this study has led to the identification of the major cardiovascular risk factors—high blood pressure, high blood cholesterol, smoking, obesity, diabetes, and physical inactivity. It has also provided a great deal of valuable information on the effects of related factors, such as blood triglyceride levels, age, sex, family history, and psychosocial issues. Although the study involved primarily Caucasians, other studies have demonstrated that the major risk factors originally identified apply almost universally among other racial and ethnic groups, although the patterns of distribution may vary. In the past half century, this study has spawned approximately 1,200 articles in leading medical journals. The concept of risk factors has become an integral part of modern medical practice that has led to the development of effective treatment and preventive strategies. And just like the goose who laid the golden eggs, the data from this project continues to yield monumentally important information.

It is now clear that heart disease is but one manifestation of widespread arteriosclerosis, a condition explained above. Lack of exercise has been of special interest, because the information from Framingham and other population studies beginning around 1950 indicate that a lifelong pattern of regular exercise not only does not pose a threat to health, but rather leads to increased longevity and quality of life. We still don't fully understand why exercise counteracts arteriosclerosis, but it seems to improve multiple risk factors such as blood cholesterol fractions, the mechanical efficiency of the heart, and decreases the tendency to develop obesity and diabetes. Nevertheless, the awakening of interest in exercise seems to have triggered a worldwide tidal wave. Substantial numbers of people are now joining fitness programs, running, and bicycling. This information may even account for the apparent reduction of interest in the building and buying of one-story houses. Unfortunately, however, far too few people have adopted this lifestyle change.

But the story of exercise does not end there. During the early 20th century, patients were scrupulously confined to bed rest for three to six weeks after sustaining heart attacks. After all, was it not logical that the heart muscle be allowed plenty of time to heal? Not so. Evidence emerged from multiple objective studies after 1960 showing that physical activity within a few days after a myocardial infarction (MI) results in higher survival rates and less sustained disability. These responses seemed to result partially from the fact that inactivity produces deconditioning of all the muscles, including the heart.

Research about exercise has also been extended to long-term management after heart attacks. Individuals who continue to engage in regular exercise enjoy more favorable outcomes, including better exercise capacity, a reduced tendency for mental depression, and even reduced long-term mortality. And exercise even benefits patients suffering from severely reduced heart function, or heart failure, by increasing their physical endurance, and probably extending their lives as well.

Other than vigorously controlling these risk factors, medical management aimed at combating arteriosclerosis was quite limited until the 1980s. Since then, a steady progression of drugs has emerged which have shown that the process of arteriosclerosis can be arrested or reversed, primarily through the reduction of blood cholesterol and related substances. But none of these drugs can work in a vacuum; they must be combined with appropriate lifestyle changes for maximum benefit. Unfortunately, this fact is often overlooked.

One notable and bizarre attempt to control the arteriosclerotic process began in the 1950s with the use of *chelation therapy*. This form of treatment, despite never having been subjected to rigorous scientific study, owes its existence to misguided logic and represents one of the greatest health myths of the twentieth century. It survives, to a degree, even to this day. It will be discussed in detail later (Chapter Thirteen).

The early application of surgical techniques to combat the ravages of heart disease provides an illuminating and colorful example of medical concepts gone awry. After Herrick's work in the early 20th century, it became apparent the arteriosclerotic process caused partial retardation of blood supply to various parts of the heart which brought about reduced heart function and— importantly—recurrent chest pains, which were often brought about by exercise. The latter is termed *angina pectoris*. These pains could be so severe that they rendered almost any activity impossible. Hence, a means to restore circulation to the heart muscle was sought. This led to a series of surgical procedures aimed—again, logically—to produce increased blood flow to the deficient areas. Two of these procedures are worthy of special note.

The first surgery involved the installation of sterile talcum powder, a known irritant, into the sac surrounding the heart.[2] It was thought that the inflammation the powder induced over the heart's surface would encourage the migration of new blood vessels and thus bring more blood to combat the shortfall. Objective confirmation was never produced, but early anecdotal reports suggested that many patients experienced relief.

Another surgical operation, called mammary ligation, consisted of tying off a surface artery that carries blood to the chest muscle.[3] It was thought—again, logically—to be capable of diverting blood to the heart muscle. After this procedure had received wide acceptance, one monumental study demonstrated that pain relief, i.e., reduction of angina pectoris—often dramatic—could be achieved following either the real surgery or a sham procedure mimicking it. These results attested to the power of the *placebo effect*, which will be discussed later (Chapter Eleven). Interestingly, all such proposed surgical procedures of the era were reported in series' of glowingly anecdotal observations in which those having undergone them experienced relief of pain.

When it comes to surgical procedures, however, proof that they are effective is difficult to establish. In contrast to new drugs, comparable controls—patients receiving a sham procedure in question, with rare exceptions as noted above—are obviously impractical or unethical, so proof of efficacy must usually be established in other ways. These may include comparison between subjects receiving an operation versus those continuing on contemporary conventional non-surgical treatment. In all situations, however, increase in circulation following surgery must be demonstrated by modern techniques that are now available.

---

[2] Thompson SA and Ralsbeck MJ. *The surgical rehabilitation of the coronary cripple.* Annals of Internal Medicine. 1949;31:1010.

[3] Dimond EG, Kittle CF, and Crockett JE., *Comparison of internal mammary artery ligation and sham operation for angina pectoris*, Am. Journal of Cardiology, 5;1960: p. 483-486.

These latter techniques may include so-called "non-invasive tests" (e.g. stress testing with nuclear isotope scanning) or "invasive" study (cardiac catheterization). Historical controls—the comparison of the results with earlier surgical efforts—can also be used, but since other factors can change with time, they are considered less acceptable as valid evidence.

The landscape for surgical procedures intended to correct blood flow to the heart changed dramatically after 1967 with the introduction of coronary artery bypass surgery. This surgery employs blood vessels (arteries or veins) taken from remote locations in the body, often the legs or superficial chest wall. These vessels are then attached to the major artery (aorta) leaving the heart and connected to the smaller coronary arteries beyond the blocked locations, thus bypassing ("leapfrogging") the obstructions. This immediately increases circulation to the heart muscle with corresponding relief of symptoms. Results of this operation have been corroborated by many subsequent objective studies throughout the world. There is little question that these surgical procedures, which are constantly undergoing refinement, provide immediate relief of symptoms stemming from coronary obstructions, and this relief correlates directly with the restoration of blood flow.

But controversy continues regarding when to use these surgical procedures in overall management of this disease. This uncertainty stems partly from the rapid advancement of alternative means of management, including medical treatment (drugs and lifestyle changes) and alternative methods of opening arterial obstructions (angioplasty with stent placement). Despite all these advances, one must realize that mechanical interventions, such as surgery and catheter techniques, provide only short-term relief of obstructions. Arteriosclerosis is a systemic disease, and proper long-term management must include medication and lifestyle changes.

All this has led to the understanding that all medical research must employ rigorous objective proof, and it is mandatory that, whenever possible, studies must compare those receiving new treatments with "controls," i.e., randomly selected comparable individuals not undergoing such treatment. Showing an apparent effect resulting simply from a series of anecdotal observations of success is now considered generally unacceptable.

All the procedures employed in Brad's management, including use of an external defibrillator, constant monitoring of heart activity, performance of moving (cinematographic) X-rays, and methods of entering blood vessels to open obstructions, were developed during the past half century. Proof that these measures are effective has been established through rigorous and painstaking objective analysis of large groups of individuals. Usually, comparisons between older and newer methods of treatment are employed, along with the application of statistical analysis to allow the separation of real effects from those due to random variations. Thus science now has a solid foothold in medical care. This constitutes evidence-based medicine.

The available research also leads me to believe strongly that lifestyle modifications, if fully implemented, would virtually eradicate the presence—and the associated complications—of arteriosclerosis,[±] including heart attacks, strokes, and other cardiovascular events, which are the main killers in our society. But given the increasing levels of obesity, persistent numbers of inactive persons, and cigarette smoking, this outcome is not likely to occur, at least in the foreseeable future. Fortunately, the ongoing progress of management, as in Brad's case, saves lives and improves outcomes, but at a very high price.

[±] Arteriosclerosis is the general term for hardening (sclerosis) of the arteries and is often used interchangeably with "atherosclerosis." This latter term refers specifically to the underlying condition in which an artery wall thickens as a result of the accumulation of fatty materials (atheroma) such as cholesterol.

The message of this chapter, however, is that if the medical profession were to rely on logic, rather than hard evidence, to make management decisions, we would be still operating in considerable darkness.

☞ *Chapter Two* ☜

WHAT IS REALLY VALID: THE SEARCH FOR TRUTH

"Believe those who are seeking the truth. Doubt those who find it."

Andre Gide

As a practitioner of conventional mainstream medicine, I am frequently bemused by patients who think I am a bona fide deity and, conversely, those who think very little of me and ignore what I say. The latter group often resorts to alternative medicines—those having no proven scientific basis. Alternative treatments include food additives, vitamins, natural or herbal medicaments, and antioxidants. They also extend to such mechanical procedures as acupuncture and chiropractic treatment. But alternatives don't stop there. Too many people fall prey to outright health frauds that are, at best, a serious waste of money, or, at worst, lead to the deterioration of health and/or failure to seek timely and effective medical care.

But we conventional medical practitioners are complicit in propagating certain myths—knowingly or otherwise. Patients come to us hoping to obtain treatments that will relieve their ailments. Naturally, any improvement noted after a given medical intervention—drug or otherwise—will usually be credited to the doctor's actions. But I must admit that this conclusion is often erroneous. But why has this illusion of treatment success been held so tenaciously by people from all backgrounds and educational levels, and from ancient times to the present? I can provide two explanations. First, most individuals will improve or recover from most maladies as a result of natural body defenses without any external action whatever. Second, the placebo effect accompanies almost every treatment, meaning there is no reason to improve from a maneuver that lacks any scientific basis. This effect usually produces a powerful reaction in the brain that brings about a perceived—real or imaginary—relief of physical discomfort or lessening of symptoms. To make matters even more interesting, the conclusion that a given medical encounter caused the improvement is compounded by another fallacy, that of *post hoc ergo propter hoc* (after this, therefore, because of this). This means that one is easily seduced by the idea that an apparent result is caused by whatever preceded it. I must admit, sheepishly, that physicians often support the illusion of cure by our readiness to accept credit for any perceived success.

But are we not in an era of modern scientific enlightenment? Shouldn't all these myths have been dispelled by the passage of time and been superseded by objective science? Unfortunately, matters of personal health, as well as many related social issues, seem to halt abruptly at science's doorstep. Why? For many years I have studied the underlying causes of misconceptions I see occurring around me almost daily. By combining concepts of physical and psychological health, many of the answers have become evident.

As a practitioner of mainstream medicine, my path has been fairly straightforward. After years of studying normal human anatomy and physiology, I embarked on a detailed quest to understand a vast array of maladies. First I learned oral questioning skills that enable me to find out the nature of the complaints that prompt an individual to seek medical care. Then came the art of the thorough physical examination and the selection of appropriate tests when necessary, such as blood analysis (testing), ECG, X-rays, and others, to evaluate the structure and performance of suspect organs. After arriving at a likely diagnosis, I would then formulate a treatment plan, which could run the gamut from reassurance that the problem would resolve spontaneously to recommending prompt, vigorous therapy, all while trying to explain plainly to the patient exactly what I was thinking. In all encounters, my conclusions are usually based on the best evidence available from the results of hundreds of well-grounded, scientific studies that involve careful, objective analysis of disease manifestations and progressions, and the effect (or lack) of available treatments. This is the sequence of events which constitute Evidence Based Medicine, or EBM.

Most contemporary scientific research involves studying of groups of individuals, then employing careful statistical analysis to determine which relationships are meaningful and which are chance occurrences. This requires plain knowledge of statistical principles and their proper application. But not all problems fit neatly into well-defined pigeonholes; which means that I—as a practitioner—must exercise my best judgment based upon principles learned through background, education, and experience. In this process, physician/scientists learned very early about the dangers of generalizing from single examples, however impressive they seem, to groups of individuals suffering from seemingly similar conditions. When studying apparent relationships between environmental exposures and subsequent diseases, we also learned how easy we could be misled into concluding falsely that a given disease or outcome was actually caused by whatever happened to precede it. These and many other practical experiences have convinced me that we are gaining ground in understanding the world's health problems.

But have those of us who represent mainstream medicine gone astray in some way? As noted above, I encounter patients frequently who, in addition to—or instead of—conventional management, are resorting to alternative measures. Those same alternatives are often being touted by claims on television, in newspapers, and in tabloid magazines near the checkout counters of grocery and convenience stores. Over half these persons are also regularly consuming multivitamin tablets and other nostrums, having no idea what outcome they're expecting. All this has stimulated my curiosity and caused me to explore the effects of alternative treatments in order to evaluate not only the current knowledge of their efficacy, but also potentially dangerous interactions with conventional medications.

At the same time, new crash diets, which defy the physical laws of conservation of mass and energy, have been appearing at a dizzying pace. They are usually promoted with the guarantee that adherence will result in weight reduction of, say, twenty pounds in a month—if you don't die first.

We are all constantly inundated with media reports declaring one medical breakthrough after another—one about a new treatment, another regarding a link between an environmental exposure and a physical or mental disorder. These announcements are often later found to be misleading, or worse yet, totally false. So, given the sheer volume of misinformation that assaults us daily, I began to wonder how this came about, and how we can, as supposedly rational practitioners, react in an effort to set the record straight.

Over the past two-hundred years, the medical community has learned how many ideas and conclusions in our field have been false and resulted in errors of judgment. To a great extent, we have been able to correct these errors; as a result, we have learned much about how judgments are formed, and therefore have been able to identify and categorize recurring errors that regularly lead to erroneous conclusions. Because we have traversed this long, circuitous, and sometimes painful path, physicians are in a position to recognize clearly common fallacies.

In my attempt to understand the biases and myths around us, I have studied many psychological and scientific medical reports that have clarified many misconceptions and answered many of these questions, which will be discussed as we progress. Because of the systematic nature of these misconceptions, my curiosity has leapt the boundaries of medical science, leading me to discover that many of these principles apply to a wide variety of experiences including, among others, perceptions about gambling odds, sporting events, financial markets, and even politics.

◈ *Chapter Three* ◈

HOW AND WHY WE DEVELOP BIASES

"Faced with the choice between changing one's mind and proving there is no need to do so, almost everyone gets busy on the proof."

John Kenneth Galbraith

Although there is some overlap, the methods from which judgments are made are generally divided into two groups: those involving numerical (statistical) concepts, and those arising from conceptual (intuitive) patterns. Although the first category has been fairly well studied, it remains surprisingly poorly understood and less well accepted by the public. The second category, intuition, is far more subjective and, therefore, more likely to lead to errors, some of which can be grievous. This category is more difficult to study, but recent observations have produced evidence that may allow better recognition of these patterns and, hopefully, the prevention of mistakes.

All humans make judgments under varying degrees of uncertainty. When little uncertainty is present, such as the likely safe arrival of a commercial air flight, we can expect a successful conclusion of trip, given the infinitesimally small chances of a mishap. But most judgments are made under considerable uncertainty, and how we form these judgments is of great importance. Fortunately, the dynamics producing such decisions have been intensively studied by numerous psychologists since the seminal studies of Tversky and Kahneman in the early 1970s.[4]

Most judgments are arrived at through a process called *heuristics,* which are experience-based techniques for problem

---

[4] Tversky A and Kahneman D. *Judgment under Uncertainty: Heuristics and Biases Science,* New Series, Vol. 185 (1974), pp. 1124-1131.

solving, learning, and discovery. These methods are generally used to speed the process of finding a good-enough solution when an exhaustive search is impractical. Terms describing this method include "rule of thumb," an "educated guess," "intuitive judgment," "common sense," and "trial and error," and employs reflexive mental operations that make complex problems manageable. While this sometimes leads to accurate judgments, it often results in dangerously flawed conclusions and biases.

We will examine many of these concepts through examples of systematic biases and associated myths. Judgments resulting from intuition alone can lead not only to bad personal decisions, but also and more importantly to flawed decisions by leaders in politics and other fields. The resulting effects have resulted in global miscalculations and disasters.

HOW WE JUDGE

Judgments are generally made on the basis of two underlying principles;[5] *intuition* and *reason*. The first principle, intuition, refers to the judgments made by heuristics. The second principle indicates those arrived at through a process of careful objective evaluation, often involving numerical and statistical concepts. Because most individuals are either unaware of statistical analysis or are unwilling or unable to devote the time and effort required for rigorous analysis, they usually revert to intuition. To avoid or minimize incorrect or biased judgments arising from intuition, reason should be applied to monitor and correct, when possible, those derived from intuition alone.

An example of the dual means by which we may arrive at decisions was presented by Kahneman[6] with the following riddle:

---

[5] Kahneman D and Frederick S. Representativeness revisited: Attribute Substitution in intuitive judgment. in Heuristics and Biases. edited by Gilovich, Griffin and Kahneman, Cambridge University Press, 2002, p. 49.
[6] Kahneman D. Thinking, Fast and Slow. Farrar, Straus and Giroux, New York, 2011, p. 44.

A bat and ball cost $1.10. The bat costs one dollar more than the ball. How much does the ball cost?

If one applies intuitive logic, or makes a snap judgment, the answer would be ten cents—which is wrong. This demonstrates the inherent pitfall in applying quick and easy logic, which Kahneman calls *System One*. More careful thought, which involves more time and effort, would produce the correct answer—five cents. This latter process is termed *System Two*, which checks and verifies the accuracy of the former. If applied properly, it will be more likely to allow one to arrive at the correct answer, although not invariably.

So our first challenge is to examine the means by which we arrive at the intuitive judgments, and demonstrate the systematic flaws to which they are subject, which often result in biases. Among the processes used for intuitive reasoning, three important ones have been identified:[7] *representativeness, availability,* and *anchoring and adjustment*.

Representativeness means the substitution of an attribute that is known for one that is unknown. I would expand that category to define it as intuitive logic, meaning that what seems like a logical conclusion is derived without critical analysis or in-depth objective observation and confirmation. Twersky and Kahneman have given an example of this process in which a mythical man, selected randomly from the general population, was described as shy and withdrawn, always helpful, having little interest in people, needing order and structure, and a having passion for detail. When individuals are asked to select his specific occupation from a list—farmer, salesman, airline pilot, librarian, or physician—most people select "librarian," because it most closely represents that occupation's stereotype. While that may be the correct answer, the conclusion does not consider the *prior probability* of that occupation. This is a reason-based concept,

---

[7] Tversky A and Kahneman D. *Judgment under Uncertainty: Heuristics and Biases Science*, New Series, Vol. 185 (1974), pp. 1124-1131.

meaning that since there are far fewer librarians in the general population than say, farmers or physicians, the second principle dictates that we adjust our probability estimates lower. This method of reaching an inaccurate decision is called *insensitivity to prior probability*, and commonly leads to biased judgments.

The so-called "domino theory" is another example of representativeness, wherein during the 1960s our leadership believed that losing a single country to communism would trigger a successive progression of additional loses to this worldwide menace, similar to a series of dominos lined up in a neat row— falling one by one. Thus the dominos were substituted for the potential series of countries. This concept, while seemingly logical, was never supported by world events and thus is another flawed concept.

But I expand the concept of representativeness to include any problem that seems amenable to an intuitively reasonable or logical solution based on parallel or analogous situations of all sorts, often invoking historical precedent for their apparent validity. So called "chelation" treatment (Chapter Thirteen) provides a medical example of this phenomenon, in which it was believed that a chemical agent that could remove calcium from the body would be effective in treating "hardening" of the arteries (arteriosclerosis), which indeed is often accompanied by calcification. This hypothesis has never been confirmed, and this treatment has been discredited, although not entirely abandoned. But the obvious conclusion is that the process of calcification is a *result* of the hardening process rather than its *cause*. In medical science, seemingly logical conclusions must be subjected to rigorous objective and unbiased study. In order to accomplish this in the attempt to establish the efficacy of a new drug or method of treatment, we usually resort to the *controlled double-blind study*, which will be discussed later.

The second means of judging by intuition is through the process of *availability*. This refers to situations in which people assess the probability of an event by the ease with which instances or occurrences come to mind. For instance, a commercial airplane disaster may create an availability response. That might result in unnecessary fear of individual air travel. On the other hand, these same individuals would likely ignore riskier activities that are far more frequent but less "available" to imagination or memory. An obvious example of the latter is that of automobile travel, for the number of fatalities from auto accidents totals approximately 33,000 yearly (1.13 fatalities per 100 million vehicle miles traveled), and this renders such travel statistically far less safe per unit mile than commercial air travel, which carries a mortality rate that is approximately 60 times lower (0.019).

Even more impressive are the data related to fatalities from cigarette smoke. Approximately 440,000 persons die annually in the United States of direct inhalation of this toxic product, accounting for an average reduction of smokers' longevity by fourteen years as compared to nonsmokers. Present estimates also increase these numbers in non-smokers regularly exposed to ambient smoke (secondary smoke) by as many as 40,000-45,000 annually. Yet, at least partially because of lesser "availability" to our collective imaginations, most people are unaware of the magnitude of this problem.

Anchoring and adjustment is defined as beginning with a starting estimate, then adjusting in the direction of the likely target—the assumed true value. This method usually biases judgments in the direction of insufficient adjustment, meaning that if the anchoring, or starting, value is too low, the adjusted value will be correspondingly low. Conversely, an excessively high starting value usually results in an inappropriately high adjusted value. Department store "sale" prices are a great example of this phenomenon. The initial retail price is the anchor, and this usually results in a mentally adjusted price that is higher than that actually listed on the price tag. Thus, psychologically, one concludes s/he is getting a real "deal"—a value lower than the mentally adjusted one. On the other hand, if there were only one price listed that was the same as the "marked down" price, anchoring would start at this lower price, the psychological effect would be reduced, and the "deal" would seem less appealing. The fact that we are constantly exposed to "sales" leads one to conclude that store owners are fully aware of this bias.

Another example of anchoring and adjustment is *hindsight bias.* In this case, when confronted with the outcome of an event, it becomes the anchor. Under these conditions, adjustment is almost never sufficient to eliminate bias in the direction the outcome should have predicted. This will be discussed in greater detail later.

An additional bias is the *confirmation bias.* This is the tendency to seek or interpret evidence favorable to pre-existing beliefs, and to ignore or reinterpret evidence that is unfavorable. This bias is formed when an initial judgment is already present. In a comprehensive review of this subject, Nickerson,[8] a psychologist, concluded that "If one were to attempt to identify a single problematic aspect of human reasoning that deserves attention above all others, the confirmation bias would have to be among the candidates for consideration." He further stated that "it appears to be sufficiently strong and pervasive that one is led to wonder whether this bias, by itself, might account for a significant fraction of the disputes, altercations, and misunderstanding that occur among individuals, groups, and nations."

Most of us harbor preconceived judgments about almost everything, and we know that almost everyone is loath to surrender or change his/her original judgments. But what compounds this problem further is the alacrity with which most people choose arguments or characteristics that support their preconceived

---

[8] Nickerson RS. *Confirmation Bias: A ubiquitous phenomenon in many guises.* Review of General Psychology. 1998;175:175-220.

notions while simultaneously rejecting those that contradict them. To confirm this concept, one need look no further than the dynamics of racial or gender bias. In this instance, the prejudged expectations of a group's characteristics lead one to evaluate a member of that group according to those expectations.[9]

In the political and economic arena, this bias applies nicely to one's willingness to accept the reality of global warming. Although all existing objective information points to real warming as a robust scientific fact, how many times do we encounter someone who denies this obvious truth—especially for political or financial gain? These attackers might simply pick out a single cold day or cold season as *confirmation* that global warming is a myth.

Confirmation bias extends to medical and scientific endeavors as well. Regarding medical conditions, hypochondriacs interpret every ache and pain as an indication of their next great health calamity, while normal people ignore them as minor random bodily signals.[10] Those suffering from psychological depression tend to focus on events and information that further reinforce the depression, and suppress evidence that things are getting better.[11]

Scientists and medical practitioners are also constantly plagued by confirmation bias. In the early days of medicine, this bias probably played a major role in the persistence of such irrational practices as bloodletting (Chapter Seventeen). In contemporary times, the pervasiveness of this bias is demonstrated by the need to perform double-blind research studies, in which both the scientists and recipients involved are shielded from the

---

[9] Hamilton DL, Dugan PM, and Trolier TK. *The formation of stereotypic beliefs: further evidence for distinctiveness-based illusory correlations.* Journal of Personality and Social Psychology. 1985;48:5-17.

[10] Pennebaker JW. And Skelton JA. *Psychological parameters of physical symptoms.* Personality and Social Psychology Bulletin 1978; 4; 524-530.

[11] Beck AT. *Cognitive therapy and the emotional disorders.* New York International Universities Press, 1976.

biases stemming from preconceived notions about the disease or treatment in question.

In conclusion, humans deal with uncertainty in various ways that often lead to biases. As noted above, judgments relying on numerical or statistical concepts are by far the most effective for problem solving, but numeric analysis is not always available. Moreover, even when numerical answers are accessible, individuals often fail to understand or overlook them and resort to intuitive problem solving, which opens the floodgates to erroneous conclusions. These errors include such concepts as failure to consider base rates, regression to the mean, and the use of insufficient numbers to form generalizations—subjects to be covered below. As a rule, individuals with statistical training are less apt to succumb to these errors, but even they are not totally immune.

✑ *Chapter Four* ✑

NUMBERS—DISTINGUISHING CHANCE FROM REALITY

"Statistics may be defined as a body of methods for making wise decisions in the face of uncertainty"

W.A. Wallis

Most people understand the meaning of a random occurrence. For instance, if we flip an ordinary coin, we would expect it to come up heads half the time. On the other hand, if the result is heads for five consecutive tosses, is this random—or something else? Simple statistical analysis says that half, or 0.5, of our first tosses will be heads. If this happens, a second straight toss will also yield 0.5 heads, meaning the chances for two consecutive tosses of heads would be half of a half (0.5 times 0.5, or 0.25). Thus there is a 25% chance we'll flip two heads in a row. This would not raise any eyebrows, and most individuals would consider it chance, or luck.

However, if we obtain the same result for five straight tosses, what is the conclusion? Applying the same mathematics, we come up with a chance of 3.1% (0.031). This means the chances of flipping heads five consecutive times are less than one in twenty (5%). These chances diminish by 0.5 with each additional roll. Thus the odds favoring 10 successive rolls of heads drop to about 0.001, or 0.1%. Could that happen? Sure, but only in about one out of a thousand runs of ten tosses. Nevertheless, the chance of heads coming up on any given upcoming individual toss remains at 50%, no matter what preceded it.

This latter point forms the basis for the gambler's fallacy— the belief there is a mysterious force that insures the odds will balance out—often driving us to double up when losing games of chance. This is also referred to as *chance has no memory.* Examples of this fallacy are profuse at the gambling casino, explaining such statements as a crap table is "hot" as a result of a shooter throwing multiple successive passes (winners). Unfortunately, this means he has won each time with each initial chance of success approximating about 50%. This form of highly flawed intuitive reasoning explains the temptation for an individual to enter any game considered "hot."

We encounter the same fallacy in other fields, notably in sports. Basketball provides a very interesting example, for there is an almost universal belief that one should get the ball to the "hot" shooter, i.e. a player who has scored baskets in rapid order within a short time. Coaches and fans alike subscribe to this doctrine. To confirm the pervasiveness of this sentiment, I quote the results from a survey of basketball fans:[12] A questionnaire was given to one hundred fans regarding sequential dependence among shots. Considerable agreement was found, for 91% of the respondents believed that a player has a better chance of making a shot after having just made his last two or three shots than he does after having missed a similar number of shots. Predictably, the majority also believed a player had a better chance of making a free throw after making the first of two than he had after missing the first shot. Is there a real statistical basis for these beliefs? We shall review the objective evidence below taken from the same source noted above:

Field goal records of nine individual players were obtained for forty-eight home games of the Philadelphia 76ers and their opponents. Surprisingly, in comparison with each player's overall hitting percentages, the chances of each one's hitting shots after one, two, or three successive hits actually fell below their seasonal

---

[12] Gilovitch T, Vallone R, and Tversky A, The hot hand in basketball: on the misperception of random sequences, in Heuristics and Biases.edited by Gilovich, Griffin and Kahneman, Cambridge University Press, 2002.p. 601.

percentages. Also contrary to expectations, their percentages were either the same or higher after missing a similar number of shots. These researchers delved deeper into the number of clustered "runs" (two or more hits in a row) for each player and found the number of these runs showed no significant statistical difference from the number expected by chance. Of course additional factors could have influenced these results, such as the amount of defensive pressure put up by the opposing team on a so-called "hot shooter" or by a possible tendency for this shooter to put up more difficult shots after feeling a surge of overconfidence after one or two successful shots. To eliminate these possible sources of inaccuracy, this study was extended to evaluate free throw percentages, and there was no evidence that success or failure of a first free throw had any influence on the second shot. Finally, they conducted experiments wherein college varsity players shot successively from controlled distances in the absence of defensive pressure, and the results were exactly the same as noted above.

How can we account for the prevalent belief in streak shooting despite the contrary results noted above? The authors of this study have presented the most likely possible mechanisms: A memory bias could have caused this illusion, because if long sequences of hits are more memorable ("available") than alternating sequences, the observer is likely to overestimate the correlation between successive shots. Careful study has confirmed that most observers "see" a positive serial correlation in randomly occurring independent sequences, and they fail to detect a negative serial correlation in alternating (also random) sequences. This holds true regardless of whether sequences are displayed to the observer in real time or retrieved from memory. The authors then state that these sequences are no different statistically from those found in coin tossing. In contrast to the coin example (admittedly random), however, since basketball is considered a game of skill, most observers prefer to believe that the encounter with successive hits was more than could have occurred by chance alone. It is highly likely that similar biases are present in other sports and endeavors, although not as carefully studied.

The authors conclude with the following statement about basketball: "If the present results are surprising, it is because of the robustness with which the erroneous belief in the 'hot hand' is held by experienced and knowledgeable observers. This belief is particularly intriguing because it has consequences for the conduct of the game. Passing the ball to the player who is 'hot' is a common strategy endorsed by basketball players and coaches. It is also anticipated by the opposing team which can concentrate on guarding the 'hot' player. If another player, who is less 'hot' on the particular day, is equally skilled, then the less guarded player would have a better chance of scoring. Thus the belief in the 'hot hand' is not just erroneous, it could also be costly."

More complex statistical analysis is used regularly in the biological and medical sciences to determine the likelihood that a given finding is real and not the result of chance biologic variation. For instance, we may use a new drug to treat 100 individuals with a given illness and find the illness is resolved in 90%. On the other hand, a similar 100 are given no treatment—a placebo—and the illness resolves in 80%. Statistical methods[#] are then used to determine the likelihood this difference in improvement could be due to the new treatment as opposed to chance, or random variation, which would suggest that the new treatment might not be effective. Employing such analysis in this example, we find the chance that random variation could account for the difference in our two groups (treated vs. untreated) is slightly above 7%. But in most medical applications, this result must be 5% or less to be generally considered a real effect, meaning the treatment is effective, although with some reservations. In example above, we do not meet the under 5% requirement for "proof"; therefore, if we wish to pursue the matter further, we might need to obtain more

---

[#] Fisher's Exact test.

convincing evidence in other settings or in other ways. The developer of this proposed new treatment might then need to decide if, based on this small preliminary sample, a next step would be warranted, such as a full clinical trial of, say, 10,000 individuals—a costly proposition indeed.

꒰ৎ *Chapter Five* ৎ꒱

**REGRESSION TOWARD THE MEAN—ANOTHER CAUSE
OF ILLUSION**

*"Say you were standing with one foot in the oven and one foot in
an ice bucket. According to the percentage people, you should be
perfectly comfortable."*

Bobby Bragan

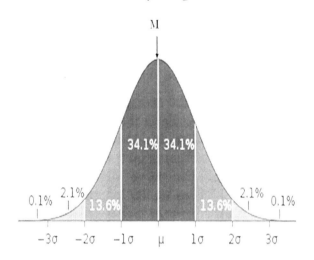

**FIGURE 1
NORMAL DISTRIBUTION (BELL) CURVE**

This picture represents how in probability theory, the so-called "normal" distribution is represented as a continuous distribution of numerous data points that has a bell-shaped configuration, known as the *Gaussian function* or informally the *bell curve*. The mean (M), or average, is at the center of this curve. The population falling within this curve is divided into sectors; each sector contains a percentage of the entire population, which is placed accordingly. At both extremes of the

41

curve are additional marks that denote the percentages of the population falling outside these limits, which are referred to as *outliers.*

Many characteristics, such as population heights and weights, can be plotted on a graph such as this. The frequency of a given measurement is generally plotted on the vertical axis, and the actual values on the horizontal axis. The result is usually a normal distribution, or bell curve. The area in the middle is where the greatest frequency of a given characteristic is found, and it represents the mean, or average, of all the values. For instance, if one were to plot the individual heights of a large population of males, the pattern would yield a bell curve, with the average (mean) height in the middle. That area would contain the greatest number of individuals.

In the United States, the average height of males is 5 feet, 9.5 inches. This mean would lie in the middle of the curve—the highest point. As the plotted heights diverge from the mean (higher or lower than 5 feet, 9.5 inches) in both directions, the number of individuals lessens, and the curve dips. At both extremes, approximately 5 feet, 0 inches on the left and 6 feet, 8 inches on the right, the curve is even lower, which is consistent with the very few persons having these measurements. The same type of curve would be produced from a multitude of other values, both medical and non-medical. Although most plots of variables result in this bell curve, some variables do not, and these extend beyond the scope of this discussion.

The concept of "regression toward the mean" is often misunderstood. In statistics it simply means, that if a variable is extreme on its first measurement, it will tend to be closer to the mean (average) on a second measurement.

For instance, if one were to observe a random group of men filing into a theater, a very short man would usually be followed by a taller one (closer to the mean), and conversely, an exceptionally tall man would usually be followed by a shorter one (again closer to the mean). This is usually true because there are far more men bunched in and around the mean value of 5 feet nine and one half than those located further out toward either end of the spectrum.

Now let us apply this concept to potential misunderstandings occurring all around us—almost daily: This concept applies readily to golf scores. A professional golfer may have an average score of 72 as opposed to a more highly ranked player, say 69. Very often at the end of the first day of a four day tournament, however, one finds a relatively low ranked player residing at the top of the leader board. Yet by the end of the fourth day, he is frequently nowhere to be found. Why this often occurs is not necessarily related to intuitive factors such as "too much pressure" or "inexperience." By the later days of the tournament, the lesser player is probably simply showing "regression" toward his particular "mean" (a higher score), whereas the higher ranked player is doing likewise when he gets better later results.

The example of tennis (or other competitive sports) is even more intriguing, for in this instance, numerical values do not apply. Nevertheless, in virtually every tennis tournament, one encounters "upsets" wherein a low ranked player beats one with a higher overall rank during the tourney. But as the tourney progresses, this same lower ranked player is very often eliminated—again because he has "regressed toward his mean" performance. Thus it is exceptional to see such a player actually winning the tourney.

Another example in personal interactions may produce misleading results. Let's use the example of a football coach who wishes to settle on the most effective strategy—reward or punishment—for achieving optimum performance of his players. Let us assume they begin by playing a great game—smashing their opponents by a large margin. As a reward, he praises their performance and gives them a day off from practice. Unfortunately, they play the next game poorly, leading the coach to conclude that reward was an inadvisable strategy, although they are actually regressing toward their "mean" performance. On a subsequent occasion, they may play extremely poorly, and as a result, the coach punishes them by increasing practice time and berating them repeatedly. What comes next, i.e., improvement to make a better showing, is highly likely and explainable by regression to their mean performance. The coach, however, not realizing the concept of regression, wrongly concludes punishment is far more effective than reward and then gauges his future behavior accordingly. This concept is easily applicable to all sorts of behavior, such as school examination scores, competition in all types of sports and contests, etc.

In medical matters, regression is commonly encountered. For instance, a given illness may fluctuate in severity around a mean level. If we happen to administer a treatment during its greatest intensity and find that it later seems recede toward a milder—mean—intensity, we are apt to be misled into the false belief that the treatment accounted for this apparent improvement rather than simple regression.

◢ *Chapter Six* ◣

INDUCTIVE REASONING AND SAMPLE SIZE— PITFALLS

"Torture numbers, and they'll confess to anything."

Gregg Easterbrook

FALLACIES OF INDUCTIVE REASONING

Inductive reasoning refers to the progression from particular individual instances to wider generalizations A generalization (more accurately, an *inductive generalization*) proceeds from a premise based upon a small sample to a conclusion about the population.

Let's assume you pick up a newspaper and read about two murders in your area, what generalizations can you make from the information? None, really. Many individuals, however, would likely conclude there was a general safety issue in the area, or that the nation as a whole is becoming less safe. Such unwarranted conclusions can often be explained by the availability bias, accounting for the failure to consider the average number of murders occurring over a longer period.

Psychologists tell us that most people tend to overgeneralize from sample sizes too small from which to derive sound conclusions.[13] Many people seem to understand the dangers of overgeneralization as reflected by the common statement, "You can't judge a book by its cover." The majority, however, seem to want to make wider generalizations. As a rule, persons with an

---

[13] Gilovitch, T. and Savitsky K., *Like goes with like: The role of representativeness in erroneous and pseudo-scientific beliefs.* in Heuristics and Biases edited by Gilovich, Griffin and Kahneman, Cambridge University Press, 2002. p. 617.

understanding of statistics are better equipped to place this concept in a more realistic perspective.

A related shortcoming of inductive reasoning is the commonly encountered *insensitivity to sample size*.[14] In this instance, small samples are thought to be representative of larger ones in that the smaller sample is expected to have the same degree of variability as the larger one. Tversky and Kahneman[15] presented an interesting example with the following riddle: "A certain town is served by two hospitals. In the larger hospital about forty-five babies are born each day, and in the smaller hospital about fifteen babies are born each day. As we know, about 50 % of all babies are boys, but this figure varies from day to day. For a period of one year, each hospital recorded the days on which more than 60 % of the babies born were boys. Which hospital do you think recorded more such days?" Interestingly, the authors found that most individuals judged the probability of obtaining more than 60 % boys to be the same in the small and in the large hospital, presumably because these events are described by the same statistic and are therefore equally representative of the general population. These authors conclude: "Sampling theory entails that the expected number of days on which more than 60 % of the babies are boys is much greater in the small hospital than in the large one, because a large sample is less likely to stray from 50 %. This fundamental notion of statistics is evidently not part of people's repertoire of intuitions." This example again demonstrates the general need to consider statistical principles in preference to intuitive conclusions whenever numerical ones are available.

Anecdotes—the use of one or a small number of individual stories, often colorful, demonstrating points of general interest—

---

[14] Kahneman D and Frederick S. *Representativeness revisited: Attribute Substitution in intuitive judgment.* in Heuristics and Biases. edited by Gilovich, Griffin and Kahneman, Cambridge University Press, 2002, p.49.

[15] Tversky A and Kahneman D. *Judgment under Uncertainty*: in Heuristics and Biases *Science*, New Series, 1974; 185:1124-1131.

are another example of flawed inductive reasoning. When used appropriately, anecdotes can add spice or humor to a presentation or exemplify or support a generally accepted principle to show how it plays out in the real world. Unfortunately, however, these stories are often misused in an attempt to establish a new general principle or to refute an already well-established scientific doctrine. For example, miraculous cures brought about by alternative medicines or procedures may be presented by individuals who have received and "swear by" such treatments, or by a television host who may be a physician benefitting from public aggrandizement, financial support, or both. These anecdotes are presented as clear evidence of a new phenomenon, or in support of a treatment of questionable efficacy despite the lack of scientific proof.

Controlled experiments involving many subjects, not anecdotes, are necessary to provide us with statistical proof. When this is not possible, experimental designs can be constructed to prospectively establish validity, often through the use of double-blind observations. In any case, never be persuaded by a single story no matter how convincingly or deftly presented.

STATISTICAL VERSUS PRACTICAL SIGNIFICANCE

One notoriously misunderstood concept is that of relative versus absolute risk reduction. The *relative risk* is a ratio of the probability of the event or disease occurring in the exposed or treated group versus a non-exposed (untreated) group. By contrast, *absolute risk reduction,* or risk difference, is the decrease in risk of a given exposure or treatment in an *overall population* in relation to a control activity or treatment.

For example, let's assume that 2% of all individuals exposed to factory smoke will experience some respiratory distress. However, if the air is filtered, the undesirable effects occur in 1%. Since the percentage has dropped from two to one, we could conclude that we have reduced this problem by 50%, meaning the *relative risk* has been halved.

But suppose we state the same data another way—the *absolute risk* has been reduced only 1%, (from 2% before, and 1% after). This is a far less impressive number. In order to create the greatest general (and emotional) impact, which way will these results most likely be reported? You guessed it—as a 50% reduction.

But if we switch to a starting rate of 50% and reduce the incidence by the same absolute 1% with air filtering, there is now a relative reduction of only 2% (50% to 49%)—hardly worth a report.

The same concept concerns the use of ordinary household aspirin, which has been found to be an excellent means to prevent heart attacks. As noted in Chapter One, these events are caused by blood clots obstructing flow through a diseased coronary artery. This means individuals who are at greatest risk for these problems are those who possess the greatest extent of this hardening process.[*] Aspirin is effective because it reduces the chances for such blood clots to occur, even when taken daily in small quantities. From a large double blinded controlled study involving 22,000 adult males, aspirin reduced the heart attack rate by approximately 45%, and subsequent studies have supported these numbers and have also shown that the rate of such attacks in women can be reduced by about 25% or more.[16] These "relative" reductions appear to hold for most prior risk categories. But how do these numbers translate into the real world, and how do these

---

[*] For enumeration of risk factors and their control the reader is referred to the American Heart Association website http://www.americanheart.org.

[16] Berger JS, Roncaglioni MC, Avanzini F., et al. *Aspirin for the primary prevention of cardiovascular events in women and men: A sex-specific meta-analysis of randomized controlled trials.* Journal Am. Med. Assoc. 2006; 295; 306-311.

"relative" reductions compare with "absolute" reductions? Let us assume a man who is fairly young and lives a lifestyle shown to keep him at low risk (non-smoker, careful diet, regular exercise, etc.) has a low approximate risk for heart attack of 1% over the next ten years. By taking regular aspirin as noted above, a person in this category could reduce his risk by 45%, that is, from 1% to 0.55%. Without going into the math, this means to prevent just one heart attack, 175 individuals in this category would need to be taking aspirin regularly over a period of ten years. From the individual's standpoint, his "relative" risk would be lowered by 45%, that is, from one in one hundred to 0.55 in one hundred, but in absolute terms, this reduction only amounts to 0.45%. In general, it is unwise for someone in this group to be taking regular aspirin because the risks of side effects to the aspirin outweigh its small potential benefits. On the other hand, let's take a male with many risk factors, possibly a smoker who is overweight with high blood pressure and diabetes. This individual may have a 20% chance of such an attack within the next ten years. Using this as a starting, or base rate, we would also expect aspirin to lower his risk by a relative 45% that is, from 20% to 11%, representing an absolute 9% reduction. Using similar numerical manipulations, this means that to prevent one attack, only ten individuals with this type of risk would need to be taking aspirin. With this background then, according to current medical guidelines, males who have a ten-year-risk greater than 6%, and women, greater than 10%, aspirin should be considered. In both genders, however, individual factors may influence the decision: these include coexisting medical conditions, kidney function, etc. Although these data cited pertain to heart disease, similar observations have been made in conjunction with certain types of strokes, i.e., sudden obstruction of diseased arteries supplying the brain. In most instances, decisions should be made with the approval of one's personal physician.

Data derived statistically from large-group studies may be misleading, or provide little or no practical guidance. A recent example of potentially misleading information based upon this type of misunderstanding stemmed from a medical report entitled "Coffee, Caffeine, and Risk of Depression Among Women."[17] In this study, researchers followed over 50,000 women for ten years and found that consumption of one or more cups of coffee daily was associated with reduced chances of mental depression developing during that period. This finding seemed to convey the impression that any given women could simply prevent depression by drinking a modest amount of coffee daily. These data were clearly valid statistically, but did this study provide any real guidance for the individual? Not really. Let's look at the actual numbers: Of the entire study population (50,739), the number developing depression over ten years was only 5.1% (2,607). Of those drinking less than one cup daily, 5.54% displayed depression versus 4.9% of those drinking more than this amount—a "relative reduction" of 11.6%. But even if coffee actually did prevent depression (which remains unproven), this means that one's actual, or "absolute," chances of warding off depression with coffee is less than one in one hundred (0.6%). Thus, from my viewpoint if I weren't especially fond of this beverage, I wouldn't start to consume it to improve my mental hygiene.

The underlying message from these examples is simple; when encountering reports of percentage changes, pay special attention to the starting percentages. The changes, however seemingly impressive and statistically valid, may have no practical meaning or application. This often involves media reports about health based on information derived from large, statistically valid studies. This may clarify why the results may have no practical worth, even when coming from apparently legitimate scientific medical sources.

---

[17] Lucas M, Mirzaei F, Pan A, et. al. *Coffee, Caffeine, and Risk of Depression Among Women.* Arch. Intern. Med. 2011; 17:1571-1578.

✐ *Chapter Seven* ✐

THE MEANING OF POSITIVE AND NEGATIVE TEST RESULTS

"I always find that statistics are hard to swallow and impossible to digest. The only one I can ever remember is that if all the people who go to sleep in church were laid end to end they would be a lot more comfortable."

Mrs. Robert A. Taft

At a recent social gathering, I encountered an acquaintance in his mid-forties who looked both fearful and upset. When I asked what was troubling him, he told me that his doctor said, after he'd undergone a treadmill stress test that he'd "flunked"—the result was "positive"—meaning to him that he was now a certified carrier of heart disease. When I questioned him further, he stated that this test was ordered as part of a routine checkup, and he'd never been told that he had heart trouble nor had he had any symptoms. He went on to say that his lifestyle was fairly "clean," meaning that he was not overweight, ate a reasonable diet, he exercised regularly, did not smoke, and was apparently free of diabetes and high blood pressure.

I then asked how he performed on the treadmill. He stated he was able to continue for at least ten minutes and, outside of being a little breathless, he felt OK. Further discussion disclosed his main concern—this test result signified impending doom. Since I did not know all his medical information, I was unable to give him a definitive answer, but I could reassure him that his positive result probably did not indicate the presence of heart disease. After further reflection, I realized how the average individual could benefit by learning about the meaning of positive results and negative results.

Almost everyone undergoes some form of medical testing, usually performed with the goal of detecting some abnormal characteristic. For example, heart disease can often be detected with stress (treadmill) testing and breast cancer with mammography. Testing extends outside the medical areas, however, as exemplified by airport security screening.

Nearly all methods of detection employ means that are not 100% accurate, meaning any given test will not detect everyone with a given condition or disclose negative findings in everyone without the same condition. Thus, we must constantly assess the chances for a certain disease to be present after a given test result is either positive or negative.

To answer these questions, we first turn to Reverend Thomas Bayes (1702–1761), an English clergyman who happened to be a fine mathematician, which was undoubtedly his first love.[18] He formulated a theorem bearing his name, which allows the mathematical calculation of probabilities of outcomes given certain baseline population characteristics. (The term *theorem* is defined as a mathematical statement that is accepted as a demonstrable truth. It should not be confused with *theory*, which will be discussed later). Bayes's formula remains pertinent and is used by contemporary health professionals, psychologists, economists, physicists, and engineers.

Bayes approached this problem on a billiard table. A first ball was thrown across the table in such a way that it was likely to come to rest anywhere on the table, and from this spot a line was drawn across the table. A second ball was then thrown multiple times, and the number of times it came to rest on either side of the line were labeled either successes or failures. By using this physical model, he calculated the probability between the two outcomes and was thus able to derive a formula.

---

[18] Bellhouse, D.R. The Reverend Thomas Bayes: a biography to celebrate the tercentenary of his birth (with discussion). *Statistical Science.* 2004; 19: 3 – 43.

The idea that Bayes introduced was *conditional probability*, i.e., the likelihood of an event occurring given that another event has already occurred. In medical issues, Bayes' Theorem usually provides a mathematical means to derive the actual probability of a disease after a given test is applied.

For example, let's return to flying for this example. We've already noted that this form of travel is approximately sixty times safer than car travel. So why are so many of us afraid of airplanes? The answer can be described in terms of conditional probabilities. The probability of dying in an air fatality is the product of two different probabilities—the probability the airplane will crash, and the probability that, in the event of a crash, the passenger will die. The first probability is extremely low—virtually zero. The second probability is one (100%)—that the individual person will die if there is a crash—and that's the probability that scares people. But according to Bayes's concept, the chance of mortality is a result of the product of these two variables—the chance of a crash times the chance of death. So, when the multiple is calculated—nearly 0 times 1—the answer is nearly zero. That is conditional probability.

Figure 2 demonstrates a pictorial version of Bayes Theorem. It shows that when a test is administered to a mixed population (some persons with and some without a given condition), it will correctly identify that condition in the majority of instances. But there are a number of misses, meaning that some individuals with the condition will have a negative (false negative) result, and some persons without that condition will register a positive (false positive) result.

In clinical medicine, we usually encounter either a positive or a negative result, and from these results, we evaluate the likelihood a given individual does or does not have the disease in question,[¥] which allows us to calculate these likelihoods based

---

[¥] Bayes' formula with an example is given in the appendix.

upon the two important factors: 1) The accuracy of the test[±] ("sensitivity" and "specificity") and 2) The composition of the population undergoing the test ("pre-test probability"). Since most tests are reasonably accurate, the most important factor in this calculation is the composition of the population being tested, i.e., the percentage already possessing the disease in question. What actually happens then, if one is testing a population containing a low rate of a given disease, a "positive" test result will usually contain a large percentage of individuals that do not have the disease in question, i.e., they are "false positives." Despite these limitations, Bayes' principle allows us to raise the likelihood of disease after a positive result and, conversely, to lower it after a negative result.

For example, let's return to treadmill stress testing. If we test a group of non-symptomatic individuals without known risk factors, it will contain a very low likelihood (pre-test probability) of heart disease—perhaps less than 1%. According to the Bayesian formula, a positive test result will still carry a low likelihood of actual disease, probably only 4% to 8%. This minimizes the practical value of this test, and under these circumstances, it will often not be recommended. On the other hand, if we decide to test an individual who has lots of risk factors combined with symptoms that indicate a higher probability of heart disease, we've raised the pre-test probability of disease to the intermediate level—possibly 50% or more. A positive test outcome in this type of individual has greater practical value, for it may raise the odds of disease to a level exceeding 90%. This then allows us to evaluate further on a much more selective basis, which is more efficient and cost-effective. Thus Bayesian principles, used daily in medical practice, allow us to better select which tests to use and how to better interpret the results.

[±] See appendix for explanation.

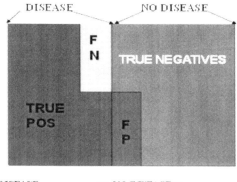

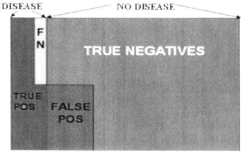

FIGURE 2

Pictorial description of the Bayes principle. We test a general population (outside box), some with a condition (Disease) and some without it (No Disease). We apply a hypothetical test to representatives from these overall populations and obtain a number of positive test results—areas labeled True Pos and FP (false pos)—and, similarly, a group of negative results—areas labeled True Negatives and False Negatives (FN). In the example at the top, half of the tested population has preexisting disease. Note that of positive responders, most have the condition (True Positives, TP), but a few do not (False Positives, FP). Conversely, of the total with negative test results, most are without the condition (True Negatives, TN), but a few have the condition (False Negatives, FN). In the example at the bottom, using the same test, we test a population with a low prevalence of preexisting disease. Note that, within this group, a positive test result contains a relatively large percentage of false positives, meaning a positive response must be interpreted cautiously. On the other hand, a negative test result contains very few false negatives (FN), meaning that a negative response weighs fairly heavily against the presence of disease.

Let us now turn to another illustrative contemporary medical situation where this type of analysis is important, that of X-ray mammography screening for detection of breast cancer. If we evaluate a population of women between ages thirty to forty, current estimates place the prevalence of cancer at approximately 1%, which is obviously quite low. We know the approximate accuracy of mammography. So given those test characteristics and such low pre-test population figures (1%), we apply Bayes formula, and what do we come up with? If a woman tests positive, the likelihood she has cancer is raised from 1% to a post-test likelihood of only 11.2%. On the other hand, however, what reassurance does a negative result provide? Applying the Bayes formula again, we now come up with a result of 99.7%, that is, the likelihood she does not have cancer. For all practical purposes, therefore, she has little or no chance of having this disease. Thus, given these underlying numbers, a negative result is far more useful and reassuring than is a positive result.

These numbers help to explain why so much controversy surrounds the issue whether widespread screening of younger women with mammography should be undertaken. Since almost 89% of positive responders will have no disease, this could potentially lead to considerable anxiety and further testing (additional imaging and/or biopsies) that entails significant expense and sometimes even risk.

To make matters even more complicated, one may ask whether very early detection of cancer with mammography at any age actually translates into lower overall mortality from breast cancer. Welch[19] has offered, in a careful review, a compelling answer to this question, concluding that, in women under the age of fifty, there is insufficient evidence to support a mortality benefit stemming from regular mammography screening. Even in those beyond this age, there is little convincing data to indicate that very early detection of subtle abnormalities—when found in individuals without palpable breast "lumps"—added any benefit in lowering ultimate mortality. Complicating matters even further, Breast cancer is a heterogeneous condition. Some tumors grow rapidly, while others grow slowly, and still others may never grow. Evaluation with a microscope cannot predict accurately with which cancer one is dealing. Thus those in the latter two categories can lead to overdiagnosis, which may be defined as "a diagnosed condition that would otherwise not go on to cause symptoms or death."[20] Mammography screening cannot distinguish between fatal and harmless breast cancer. Although exact numbers are evasive, best estimates of overdiagnosis place this percentage between 15% and 25% of all those found to have evidence of tumors in mammograms.[21] This presents a real dilemma to both patient and physician alike. Unfortunately, at this time we lack the necessary tools to reliably identify which breast cancers will be fatal without treatment and which can be safely observed over time without intervention. One possible approach would be to follow abnormalities detected with mammograms over time to detect evidence of enlargement before a surgical biopsy is performed. This would obviously be a tough sell for both women and physicians who would be fearful of missing a potentially fatal condition that might become irreversible with time. Hopefully

---

[19] Welch HG et. al. *Overdiagnosed*. Beacon Press, Boston, Mass. 2011, p.73-89.

[20] Elmore JG. And Fletcher SW. Overdiagnosis in breast cancer screening: Time to tackle an underappreciated harm. Ann. Int. Medicine. 2012;156:536-537.

[21] Kalager M, Adami HO, Bretthouer M, Tamimi RM. Overdiagnosis of invasive breast cancer due to mammography screening: results from the Norwegian screening program. Ann. Inter. Med. 2012;156:491-499.

better methods will be available in the near future to resolve this pressing issue.

As already illustrated, if we increase the pre-test odds of cancer by additional factors such as a strong family history or the discovery of a suspicious lump in the breast on physical examination, then a positive mammogram carries a much higher probability of cancer; moreover, it likely offers a much greater chance of increasing survival from this disease, again thanks in part to Reverend Bayes.

Although of tremendous importance in clinical medical practice, where it is used daily, Bayes's concept also applies interestingly to many other situations, even those that do not involve numerical calculations. In an earlier section (see Chapter Three), we described an individual taken at random from the general population that seemed to match that of a stereotypical librarian. One's subjective interpretation of the likelihood that this description would actually be that of a librarian must be tempered by the "base rate" of librarians in the general population. Thus, if this base-rate of librarians were perhaps only two or three percent of the population at large, the subjective estimate may only raise this likelihood only modestly, perhaps to a level of only ten or twenty percent. Therefore, despite an intuitive description match, such a given individual would still be unlikely to be a librarian.

Bayes's concept also applies interestingly to other non-medical situations such as airport screening. Even if the various preliminary screening devices had a very high accuracy (probably a specificity of greater than 99%), the fact the groups subjected to this screening have such an infinitesimally small rate of dangerous or explosive devices, then a "positive" test response will almost certainly be a "false positive." This conclusion is clearly confirmed by the monotonous regularity with which no real threats turn up in response to the secondary screening methods, i.e., "wanding," pat-downs, etc. I suspect that if Reverend Bayes were here today, he would be both surprised and gratified by the worldwide acceptance of his theorem, except when he would need to undergo a "pat-down" prior to entering a new-fangled airplane.

ᥱ✐ *Chapter Eight* ✎ᥩ

CONFUSION IN DETERMINATION OF CAUSES OF PAST EVENTS

"We learn from history that we never learn anything from history."

Hegel

"Some historians hold that history...is just one damned thing after another."

Arnold Toynbee

We are deluged by all types of events every day, and humans have a natural curiosity and need to explain the underlying causes. This is reasonable, because if occurrences are unfavorable or dangerous, we try to fathom their causes and avoid or prevent repeat occurrences. Having determined the likely causes, we may use this information to allow us to predict, hopefully with success, similar events in the future. But the analysis of causes of past events is fraught with pitfalls. Predicting the future is even more hazardous, especially because it often depends on the proper assessment of past dynamics.

After one is convinced we have been confronted by a real event, not just a chance occurrence, then another challenge waits. Can we account for any occurrence in any rational way that avoids many pitfalls plaguing human intuition?

Post Hoc Fallacy

Why are you standing here on this street corner?
Wildly waving your hands and shouting?
"I'm keeping away the elephants"
But there aren't any elephants here.
"You bet: that's because I'm here."

Traditional Tale

Again, the post hoc ergo propter hoc fallacy means that if an event follows another, the preceding must have caused the following. For instance, if one takes a multiple vitamin and does not catch cold, then the vitamin must have prevented all colds and possibly other assorted illnesses. Or did it?

I believe that post hoc reasoning usually does not establish the presence of cause and effect. But since many instances might really demonstrate causation, how can we make this distinction? In most situations the answer is not clear. Say we observe that a few individuals take large doses of a given vitamin and seem to catch few colds. How do we know the vitamin was responsible? Would this illness have been absent even if the vitamin were not taken?

We form a hypothesis that the vitamin might be effective in preventing the illness. To prove this, we design a double-blind controlled trial and enroll a large number of volunteers to participate. The group is divided randomly and equally into a "treated" group (given the vitamin), and a "control" group (given identical tablets that are inactive). Neither the subjects receiving, nor those administering, the tablets would know who was receiving the active tablets. This withholding of knowledge from both groups is called *double blinding*, and it usually prevents biased results. Bias poses a two-way danger. If the subjects were to know they were receiving the placebo, they would more likely report a lack of success, in contrast to those believing they were receiving the "active" drug.

During the study, the results are usually monitored by a third party who confidentially maintains the information. After a suitable period of observation, the results are then tabulated and analyzed to ascertain whether or not the active agent reduced the incidence of colds versus the control group. If the frequency of colds is lessened, then statistical methods are employed to determine how likely this reduction could have occurred by chance factors alone. In general, if the analysis discloses a probability of less than 5%, the agent in question is generally deemed effective. Even then, the results of such individual studies are usually not considered absolute proof until other investigators in other locations confirm the results independently.

THE ENVIRONMENT AND DISEASE: ASSOCIATION OR CAUSATION?

Media reports constantly bombard us with the purported dangers of exposure to noxious outside forces, from radio waves to cell phones to all sorts of chemicals. Statisticians and epidemiologists can inform us there may be a significant correlation between an environmental exposure and a given disease, but does that mean the environmental event is the cause? Are there rules that can help us determine whether a given preceding event may actually be the cause? This question is difficult because proof of cause is seldom available. In a classic report in 1965, Hill[22] presented guidelines for assessing likely causation. He points out the following:

"There are, of course, instances in which we can reasonably answer these questions [about cause and effect] from the general body of medical knowledge. A particular, and perhaps extreme, physical environment cannot fail to be harmful; a particular chemical is known to be toxic to man and therefore suspect on the factory floor. Sometimes, alternatively, we may be

---

[22] Austin Bradford Hill, *The Environment and Disease: Association or Causation? Proceedings of the Royal Society of Medicine*, 58 (1965), 295-300.

able to consider what might a particular environment do to man, and then see whether such consequences are indeed to be found. But more often than not we have no such guidance, no such means of proceeding; more often than not we are dependent upon our observation and enumeration of defined events for which we then seek antecedents. In other words we see that the event B is associated with the environmental feature A, that, to take a specific example, some form of respiratory illness is associated with a dust in the environment. In what circumstances can we pass from this observed association to a verdict of causation? Upon what basis should we proceed to do so?"

Hill then presented a series of guidelines; the major ones are listed below in order of importance. For purposes of demonstration, they are applied to the relationship between cigarette smoking and lung cancer:

1. Strength of association—the degree to which a certain disease is increased following a given exposure. He noted that prospective inquiries established the death rate from lung cancer in cigarette smokers was nine to ten times the rate in non-smokers, and the rate in heavy smokers was twenty to thirty times than that of the base value. This would be considered to be a strong association as opposed to a twofold rise in incidence.

2. Consistency of association—whether the association has been repeatedly observed by different persons, in different places, circumstances, and times. The relationship between smoking and cancer is the same in hundreds of studies derived from a wide variety of situations and techniques. And repeated exposure to smoke in non-smokers increases their risk of cancer.

3. Specificity of association—whether a specific disease is related to a single type of exposure. Even though exposure to cigarette smoking is associated with other maladies, most notably cardiovascular disease, it is by far best correlated specifically with

lung cancer. And although lung cancer occurs in individuals lacking such exposure, it is quite rare.

4. Temporal relationship of association—whether the unfavorable outcome follows the suspected noxious culprit. Which is the cart and which is the horse? A rather far-fetched example of this would be a surprising revelation that smoking was taken up regularly in response to already established cancerous conditions.

5. Biologic gradient—whether there is a *dose-response curve*. As implied in example 1, the death rate from lung cancer rises linearly with the number of cigarettes smoked daily. This fact, in itself, is quite incriminating.

6. Biologic plausibility and coherence—the existence of other biologic evidence that supports a causal explanation. We know that exposure to agents contained in cigarette smoke can cause cancer in other organs, thus implicating the likelihood of the same effect on the lungs. Cigarette smoke has been associated with cancers in skin, urinary tract, oral and nasal cavity, esophagus, larynx, pancreas, stomach, cervix, colon, and is even related to certain types of leukemia. Moreover, cancer can be induced in laboratory animals by exposure to cigarette smoke. However, the argument for biologic plausibility is not always possible because it often depends on the experimental information available in the same era. Thus we may seek and obtain biologic confirmation in the laboratory after the fact.

7. Experimental confirmation—by intervening to eliminate the suspected offender, we can show that the disease in question is prevented or eliminated. Repeated studies have shown that cessation of smoking reduces the rate of cancer.

Hill goes on to state that statistical significance between an environmental factor and a given disease does not provide proof of causation. He cites interference by confounding factors such as selection bias or inadequate sample sizes. Finally, he considers what level of evidence might justify preventive actions. He admits, as have many others, that this complex challenge requires the consideration of such issues as the cost of interventions, the likely benefits if preventive measures are successful, and the strength of evidence supporting a causal relationship. In other words, evidence or belief that causal relationship exists is not itself sufficient to suggest taking action. Conversely, uncertainty about whether there is a causal relationship, or even an association, is not sufficient to suggest action should not be taken. Each circumstance may dictate a different response. Clearly, there are no easy answers.

We cannot escape the overwhelming evidence establishing cigarettes as a cause of lung cancer. Similar evidence, not detailed here, links smoking almost as convincingly to cardiovascular disease. Nevertheless, when bombarded by alleged relationships between other environmental exposures, the reader is cautioned not to accept them without serious skepticism. Insist at least upon confirmation from multiple sources under differing circumstances.

POST HOC PITFALLS

The relationship between female hormones (estrogen and progestin) and cardiovascular disease provides a prime example of this pitfall. Women in general suffer from a lower rate of these diseases when compared with men; however, after menopause, they become afflicted at an increasing rate and begin catching up with men. The "logical" conclusion was that female hormones— diminishing after menopause—protect against these diseases. Thus large numbers of women received hormone replacement for many years presumably for protection against such diseases. Since this original premise was based on population observations, prospective double blinded studies surprised the entire medical world, for they showed no protective effect of these hormones.[23] [24]

---

[23] Hulley S, et al., *Randomized Trial of Estrogen Plus Progestin for Secondary Prevention of Coronary Heart Disease in Postmenopausal Women. American Medical Association, 1998; 19; 280:605-13.*

Thus these hormones are wisely avoided or discontinued not only because of their lack of benefit, but also by their tendency to promote blood clotting, leading to a greater incidence of strokes (clots in blood supply to the brain) and thrombophlebitis (clots in various veins). An even more important reason to avoid hormonal use is they appear to increase the frequency of breast cancer. Recent support for this latter conclusion was supplied by a study in California where invasive breast cancer incidence rates declined 33.4% between 2001 and 2004, paralleling the dramatic reduction in hormone use during this same period.[25] Hopefully, conclusions from this latter observation will not prove to be another *post hoc* error, but that awaits confirmation from additional studies.

Yet another example of potentially dangerous conclusions stemming from the *post-hoc* fallacy is exemplified by a study published in 1999,[26] describing a small group of twelve children who were supposedly normal until after they received a standard immunization to prevent measles, mumps and rubella (MMR), presumably developing autism in the aftermath. Even if accepted as a valid observation, the numbers in this study were very small and, as noted above, careful controlled studies would have been necessary to establish a causative role for the immunizations. Nevertheless, this report ignited a worldwide scare over vaccines and autism—and caused millions of parents to delay or decline potentially lifesaving immunizations for their children. Subsequently numerous independent studies were performed and failed to find any link between vaccines and autism. Certain procedural problems uncovered after its publication casted serious doubt on the integrity of the original study. Unfortunately,

---

[24] Anderson GL at al, The Women's *health initiative randomized controlled trial*, Journal of the American Medical Association, 2004;291:1701.

[25.] Ereman RR, Prebil LA, Mockus M, et al. Recent trends in hormone therapy utilization and breast cancer incidence rates in the high incidence population of Marin County, California. BMC Public Health. 2010; 10: 228.

[26] Wakefield AJ. MMR vaccination and autism. Lancet. 1999; 354:949–950.

vaccination rates in England and worldwide plummeted after the study was publicized. To this date, nearly 40% of American parents also have declined or delayed a vaccine, according to the Center for Disease Control. Many parents now have a vague distrust of vaccines—with little to no memory of diseases that terrified their grandparents.

EVALUATION OF CAUSES EXTENDING BEYOND MEDICAL SCIENCE

Very important examples of the *post-hoc* fallacy extend to our political system with potentially dreadful results, and they are obviously not subject to experimentation or outright refutation: for instance, president G.W. Bush stated publicly that one of the major "accomplishments" of his administration was that for the seven years after the terrorist attack of September 11, 2001, there were no further major attacks by terrorists in U.S. territory, thus suggesting a direct effect by his administration on dissuading further efforts by terrorists. While this is one possibility, such a conclusion is uncertain. There were attacks during the same period in Europe and Asia: Are we to conclude that administrations in other countries were less vigilant or effective than in the U.S.? Or could it be that these nations were simply located nearer to terrorist cells, permitting easier access to targets? Or were no attacks on U.S. soil planned by potential terrorists for any other reason? These questions and others cast considerable doubt on such a conclusion, and what may be far worse, could lead to the conclusion that some measures, such as "harsh interrogation techniques" may have brought about this apparently favorable result.

With regard to national economics, the *post-hoc* fallacy is clearly alive and well—providing ammunition for those wanting to "prove" both positive and negative outcomes. The so-called governmental "stimulus package" that was supposed to prevent and combat the severe national recession that began in 2008 is a good example. Those who were responsible for creating this package claim it is "working," for without it, the economy would have been far worse and, given sufficient time, it will eventually bring about complete recovery. Those who were critical of this effort state that the benefit of the package, if present at all, is very slow and, therefore, cannot be attributed to the government's efforts. Many of this latter group say these "stimulus" efforts are harming the economy, preventing a more rapid recovery while, at the same time, increasing the national deficit. So who is "correct" in this analysis? This question has no definite answers. If one consults the various pundits such as economists, one is likely to find opinions to support either contention. Making matters worse, those with political agendas can easily find support for their own political philosophies, demonstrating a form of confirmation bias.

Additional examples of the *post-hoc* fallacy are too numerous to mention and legendary for the damage they have wreaked throughout the world. They extend to all levels of personal experience, government and politics. When we attempt to analyze sequences in history, our ability to identify true cause and effect relationships is notoriously shortsighted and subject to inaccurate conclusions.

By contrast, at least in the case of scientific inquiry, Sagan[27] has said the following:

"Science has an overwhelming advantage over history, because in science we can do experiments. If you are unsure of the negotiations leading to the Treaty of Paris in 1814-1815, replaying the events is an unavailable option. You can only dig into old records. You cannot even ask questions of participants. Every one of them is dead. But for many questions in science, you can rerun the event as many times as you like, examine it in new ways, test a wide range of alternative hypotheses. When new tools are devised,

---

[27] Sagan C. *The Demon-Haunted World*. Ballantine Books. New York, N.Y., 1997. p. 254.

you can perform the experiment again and see what emerges from your improved sensitivity. In those historical sciences where you cannot arrange a rerun, you can examine related cases and begin to recognize their common components. We can't make stars explode at our convenience, nor can we repeatedly evolve through many trials a mammal from its ancestors. But we can simulate some of the physics of supernova explosions in the laboratory, and we can compare in staggering detail the genetic instruction of mammals and reptiles."

This review cannot provide sweeping answers to questions as to whether many specific *post hoc* conclusions are really valid, that is, capable of uncovering truly "cause and effect" situations. We merely wish to apply a healthy dose of skepticism when hearing assertions of this nature—whether by political leaders, by friends at cocktail parties, and perhaps most importantly, when the individual is tempted to draw such conclusions on a personal level.

◌ﾟ *Chapter Nine* ◌ﾟ

HINDSIGHT BIAS, OR THE MONDAY-MORNING QUARTERBACK FALLACY

"Of all the forms of wisdom, hindsight is by general consent the least merciful, the most unforgiving."

John Fletcher

Although most of us are aware of the *Monday-morning quarterback* manner of thought distortion, also referred to as *20/20 hindsight*, psychologists' studies have provided some interesting insight.[28] Once people know the outcome of an event, they not only tend to view what has happened as inevitable, but also as relatively inevitable before it happened. That means that, if asked afterwards how they would have predicted the outcome if they had held the original pre-event perspective, they believe they should have anticipated the event before it happened. Psychologists have found that individuals modify their remembered opinions prior to the event in a way that would have made anticipation of the outcome more likely. This seems related to the ease of recalling the actual outcome and integrating this recall into the before-and-after sequence. To achieve such a distortion, we must falsify our memory of the prior factors that led to the event [29]—in essence, lie to ourselves. And belief in such a distortion is so firm that de-biasing these prejudices is extremely difficult, if not impossible. In fact, the

---

[28] Fischhoff B. *For* those *condemned to study the past.* in Heuristics and Biases, ed. by Kahneman D, Slovic P and Tversky A. Cambridge University Press, Cambridge, U.K, 1982, p.422.

[29] Hawkins SA and Hastie R. *Hindsight: biased judgment of past events after the outcomes are known.* Psychological Bulletin, 107; 311-327, 1990.

findings suggest that forcing oneself to argue against the inevitability of the outcome is extremely difficult.[30]

For example, personal outcomes we feel we should have anticipated can cause considerable distress, if not outright guilt. "If only I had gone to the physician earlier, my cancer would have been detected before it had become incurable..."If I hadn't allowed my son to have used the car that night..." All of us have experienced similar episodes, and most of us find it extremely difficult, if not impossible, to comprehend in advance why we didn't understand the signs that seem to have been clear. And the list goes on and on.

But hindsight bias extends powerfully into national or political events, often with potentially disastrous consequences: for instance, after the terrorist attacks of Sept. 11, 2001, public and political criticism was leveled against many of our officials regarding why they did not properly assess the signs that could have led inevitably to the apprehension of the perpetrators prior to the actual disaster. Conventional wisdom (falsely) dictated that prevention "should have" been not only possible but accomplished.

When hindsight bias guides future behavior, the results can be even more unfavorable—if not calamitous. Politicians and historians often use the example of the events leading to the outbreak of the Second World War, saying that if the allies had "stood up" to Hitler during his earlier transgressions, we could have prevented this war entirely. Not only is this conclusion highly questionable, but it still provides a rationale for our behavior against future "Hitler-types" such as Saddam Hussein in Iraq. Regardless of the ultimate outcome in Iraq, our basis for entering this war was highly tenuous and to some extent likely attributable to this "Hitler" illusion.

---

[30] Fischhoff B. *For those condemned to study the past.* in Heuristics and Biases, ed. by Kahneman D, Slovic P and Tversky A. Cambridge University Press, Cambridge, U.K, 1982, p.422.

71

As a result of these biases, the tenacity of preconceived notions about the ability to predict future world events was well demonstrated by a psychological study by Tetlock.[31] In this study, experts in political and foreign policy were questioned before various world events unfolded about the future of the Soviet Union, South African apartheid, European Monetary Union, and survival of Canada's unity. When compared afterwards with the actual outcomes of these events, these experts demonstrated no greater accuracy than by chance. When questioned again after the events transpired, the various experts—whether proven to be correct or incorrect—showed no real changes in their underlying thought processes that might modify future approaches. Most notably, those who were incorrect responded by rationalizing their responses with such explanations as they almost got it right, there was an unexpected change in the event's timing, all the preexisting conditions were not met, or they were simply "unlucky." Although the complexity of these predictions does not lend itself to direct or simple conclusions, this does not bode well for our ability to confront future world problems with any greater accuracy than throwing darts at a board. Perhaps this confirms the various statements that we learn nothing from history.

In the sporting fields, examples of hindsight bias are too numerous to mention: "Why did the coach not call a time-out before the game-winning shot was made?" "Why was an intentional walk given to a batter before the next batter connected for a game-winning home run?" And so on.

---

[31] Tetlock PE, *Theory-driven reasoning about possible pasts and probable futures: Are we prisoners of our preconceptions?* American Journal of Political Science, 1999; 43:335-366.

⟆ *Chapter Ten* ⟇

FALLACIES IN PREDICTING FUTURE EVENTS

"Politics is the ability to foretell what is going to happen tomorrow, next week, next month and next year. And to have the ability afterwards to explain why it didn't happen."

Winston Churchill

"You can never plan the future by the past."

Edmund Burke

When dealing with past occurrences, we must determine that an event is not a result of random factors alone. If we accomplish this successfully, we are then challenged to determine the underlying causes of such events. Even more daunting, however, is the task of determining likely future outcomes. Perhaps Yogi Berra put it best when he stated, "the future ain't what it used to be."

Systematic biases usually hamper our efforts. According to psychologists, the main source of errors in predictions is probably excessive confidence in one's own ability to perform. This is closely related to excessive optimism[32] which, although not invariable, predominates. The *planning fallacy* is a useful example of this bias—people expecting to finish personal projects—such as school work or Christmas shopping—in less time than required.

When we predict likely outcomes, we usually employ recognized techniques of logic, including applying past experiences that duplicate, or at least resemble, past events to

---

[32] Armor DA and Taylor SE, *When predictions fail: The dilemma of unrealistic optimism,* in "Heuristics and Biases, The Psychology of Intuitive Judgment," edited by Gilovich, Griffin and Kahneman, Cambridge University Press, 2002, p. 334.

derive likely future outcomes. We think we can learn from past events and so must use that information lest history repeat itself. Unfortunately, historical conditions seldom, if ever, provide us with circumstances that resemble the past sufficiently to provide strict guidelines from which to draw a plan of action.

Let's return to a variation of the domino theory for an example. The conventional attitude expressing the relationship between marijuana and opiate use holds that use of marijuana (cannabis or pot) commonly, if not inevitably, leads to the use of opiates, such as morphine and heroin. More aggressive proponents suggest there is a domino effect as individuals begin their addiction with cigarettes, which lead successively to marijuana and opiates. But is there evidence for such an association?

Among confirmed opiate addicts, there is a high rate of use of marijuana, which often begins prior to narcotic use.[33] But these data are derived retrospectively from a select group likely to have underlying personality traits that cause them to seek more than one drug or experience. Also undermining the likelihood of a direct association between marijuana and opiates is the fact that their relative use is influenced by a person's environment. For instance, in metropolitan areas where drug dealers are numerous, there appears to be greater acceptance of narcotics among those who have at least experimented with marijuana. On the other hand, in many Southern states, opiate addiction is often unassociated with marijuana. And according to a recent study of people who have used marijuana at least once, they have only a one in twenty-six chance of using opiates at any time in their life. That author concludes that marijuana experimenters rarely turn to hard drugs, which is further substantiated by the fact that in general there are far more marijuana than narcotic users.

There is also a medical reason to support these contentions, and that relates to the meaning of addiction. Although still subject

---

[33] Goode E (ed) *Marijuana*, Transaction Publ, Piscataway, N.J., 2009. pp. 47-50.

to some debate, addiction can occur at two different levels—psychological and physical. Psychological addiction means individuals compulsively desire repeated exposure to a given substance for its euphoric effects, but cessation does not cause any physical symptoms of withdrawal. Physical addiction refers to a specific progression of events in which the addicting substance initially produces euphoria and pain relief (in the case of opiates). With repeated exposure, however, the body develops a tolerance—progressively increasing doses are required to produce the same level of euphoria or pain relief. After tolerance develops, stopping the drug results in uncomfortable, or even life-threatening, objective physical withdrawal symptoms. Because of this, physicians are loath to prescribe opiates for individuals suffering from chronic pain because if the underlying cause is not successfully controlled, the result may be both pain and addiction.

Among the many agents that are capable of producing this so-called tolerance/withdrawal effect are the pain-relieving drugs, which include all the opiates.$^{\infty}$ Other drugs with addictive potential include barbiturates such as phenobarbital, sodium thiopental and secobarbital; benzodiazepines such as diazepam (Valium^R), lorazepam (Ativan^R), and alprazolam (Xanax^R). This list includes also—and especially noteworthy—nicotine and alcohol. Lesser known substances also possess these features, but are not listed here. I consider this group of drugs as "vicious" offenders because they produce combined psychological and physical dependence. Of all the various substances capable of producing withdrawal symptoms, however, alcohol can produce the most dramatic. Depending upon how long one imbibes alcohol continuously, withdrawal produces a progression of abnormalities, most severe after a period of approximately six weeks or more of continuous intake. These latter manifestations include full-fledged convulsive

---

$^{\infty}$ The category of opiates includes morphine, heroin, codeine, oxycodone, buprenorphine, nalbuphine, methadone, and fentanil.

seizures, identical to those of epilepsy, and these have been known throughout antiquity as "rum fits." Delirium tremens is also part of this picture, and this condition, if not treated aggressively, can even result in death. I was rudely introduced to these pernicious outcomes during my early training at a busy general hospital in Philadelphia.[34]

Interestingly, absent from this list of physically addictive substances are the so-called "uppers" that include cocaine and methyl amphetamine. While these latter drugs may lead to some depression on withdrawal, there are no identifiable deleterious physical withdrawal effects. Also not on this list is marijuana. Thus while this latter agent has the potential to produce the psychological need for repetitive exposure, it could also be used intermittently as a "recreational" substance, and the cited data seem to support this contention. As a matter of fact, the absence of a threat to produce physical/withdrawal places marijuana in a category above that of alcohol.

Aside from recreational use, marijuana has valuable medicinal properties. Although this has been disputed, and despite the opposition to research and use put forward by national governments, it does have well-documented beneficial effects, including ameliorating nausea and vomiting in gastrointestinal illness, stimulating hunger in chemotherapy and AIDS patients, and lowering intraocular eye pressure in glaucoma patients.

My purpose in discussing this issue is to expose the biases that can arise from intuitive reasoning in which we draw inappropriate, representative parallels with other situations, such as dominos. I do not necessarily advocate legalization of marijuana, but I oppose biases that offer a doomsday scenario if we were to

---

[34] Tavel, ME. *A new look at an old syndrome: delirium tremens.* Arch Intern Med. 1962;109:129-134.

legalize it. To suppress its legalization may be as senseless as the prohibition of alcohol during the 1920s. At the time of this writing, sixteen states and the District of Columbia have legalized the possession of marijuana, and there is a growing federal movement for at least partial legalization. Tax revenues arising from legalization provide an extra incentive for governmental consent.

GENERAL FALLACIES OF PREDICTION

<u>Stock and Equities Predictions:</u> Financial markets offer excellent examples for analysis, not only for exploration of underlying psychological dynamics, but also as a means to manage—and hopefully protect—one's own assets. We have always known that financial markets overreact, especially stock prices on the various public exchanges. For instance, Shiller,[35] using the now well-known term "irrational exuberance," found survey evidence during the 1987 stock market crash that investors were overreacting to each other's behavior rather than to hard economic data. A study by De Bondt and Thaler[36] demonstrated that the mean reversion in stock prices is evidence of overreaction, that is, stocks that were extreme losers over an initial three to five year period earned excess returns over subsequent years. In a later paper, these authors showed these excess returns were best explained by negatively biased expectations of future earnings and not to changes in risk, tax effects, or other anomalies. This meant earnings recovery had outpaced the recovery in stock prices because the bias of excessive investor pessimism had interfered with the correct anticipation of this reversal in earnings.

---

[35] Shiller RJ. Irrational Exuberance, Princeton University Press, Princeton, NJ. 2000.
[36] De Bondt WFM and Thaler RH. Do analysts overreact? in Gilovitch, T. and Savitsky K., The Psychology of Intuitive Judgment. in Heuristics and Biases, edited by Gilovich, Griffin and Kahneman, Cambridge University Press, 2002, p. 678.
[37] Dreman D.,Contrarian investment strategies: The next generation. New York. Simon and Schuster, 1999.

Overall predictions of future stock prices and earnings by the general population of investors are regularly biased toward excessive optimism.[37] This optimism can be easily explained when considered against the background of the overall leaning toward positive bias exhibited by the average person, as noted above, and by numerous psychological studies. But could much of this bias result from the advice given by professionals such as security analysts? De Bondt and Thaler[36] have provided a clear answer to this question. In evaluating the performances of a large number of analysts over two years, they found these professionals' predictions of future earnings were regularly too extreme and optimistic: The actual earnings changes averaged only 65% of the forecasted one-year changes, and for their two-year forecasts, this number was even lower—46%. Moreover, the larger the forecasted changes, the larger the forecast errors. These authors also considered that analysts may have incentives to make biased forecasts to support their employers' underwriting business, but they found similar biases in areas without such potential financial incentives such as predicting future currency exchange rates and macroeconomic variables.

Extending the observations about security analysts' failures one step further, what do we know about the overall ability of general stock traders and professional investment managers to pick financial stocks successfully? Contrary to popular belief, Kahneman[38] presents cogent evidence that, with regard stock picking, both groups are highly inaccurate. Through extensive analysis, he cites evidence that, while individual investors on average regularly lose money, their results are so dismal that they actually equate with "an achievement that a dart-throwing chimp could not match." But even the so-called experts are also usually flawed. Professionals are able to predict short term outcomes and,

---

[38] Kahneman D. Thinking, Fast and Slow. Farrar, Straus and Giroux, New York, 2011, pp. 212-217.

in the process, to extract a considerable wealth from amateurs, but few stock pickers, if any, have the skill needed to beat the market consistently, year after year. Thus even the experts cannot successfully predict long-term outcomes. This adds further confirmation to the well-known fact that at least two out of every three mutual funds underperform the overall market in any given year.

Although excessive financial bias is clearly slanted toward optimism, negative bias is also common, but less extreme. This skewed effect also helps explain the relative impact of earnings "surprises" on stock prices that result from revisions of predicted earnings. David Dreman[37], a respected "contrarian" investor, observes the following: 1) Positive surprises result in major appreciation for out-of-favor stocks, while having minimal effect on favorites. 2) Negative surprises result in major drops in the price of favorites while having virtually no impact on out-of-favor stocks. What he is saying, simply stated, is the so-called "touted" stocks already have a more excessive preexisting positive bias built in before any surprise announcements. Taken as a whole, this information lends strong support to the contrarian attitude toward investing, that is, after doing one's homework, consider the out-of-favor ("beat down") stocks that continue to have strong underlying earnings performance despite excessive falls in stock price, but this may require patience. These dynamics probably also help explain movements in the markets as a whole, for it is common knowledge that markets fall much more rapidly and more severely than they rise. From these observations, the individual investor should beware that forecasted changes—especially on the positive side—are simply too extreme to be considered rational. The fact that such overreaction is exhibited by professional economists and analysts adds extra caution to what people read and how they should plan their investment strategy.

Adding further support to these conclusions about the financial markets, George Soros[39] has proposed the concept of "reflexivity," in which he explains that, contrary to conventional wisdom that markets are "always right," he believes they are actually "always wrong." By that he means they are usually either overpriced or underpriced. His explanation for this follows: Classical economic theory is mistakenly equated with physical science, that is, they should behave according to fixed principles and, as a result, should be totally predictable by outside observers. But economics is not a physical science and individuals making the predictions and economic decisions are also influencing these markets toward inordinate excesses. Thus the markets behave in a "reflex" way to these unbalancing and biased forces. These excessive biases then affect the fundamental valuations they are supposed to reflect. The resulting fundamentals may then further reinforce the biased expectations, an initially self-reinforcing but eventually self-defeating process. This theory goes a long way toward explaining the repetitive boom-bust cycles, the Great Depression, and the severe downturn that began in 2008. This also explains why, in the social or financial realm, the future can never be predicted with unerring accuracy, for if people were provided in advance with a "certain" outcome in financial markets, they would act in ways that would alter or nullify this expected outcome. This line of reasoning supports Soros' theory of reflexivity (maybe as good as Einstein's theory of relativity?)

Historical Experience as a Basis for Predictions: When we predict likely outcomes, we usually employ recognized techniques of "logic." These include applying past experiences that duplicate—or at least resemble—past events to derive likely future outcomes. We often think that we can learn from past events and, therefore, must use this information since "history often repeats itself." Unfortunately, historical conditions seldom, if ever, provide

---

[39] Soros G. *The New Paradigm for Financial Markets*. Public Affairs, New York, N.Y. 2008.

us with enough circumstances that resemble the past sufficiently to permit strict guidelines from which to draw a plan of action. We have already observed the apparent futility in trying to draw an analogy between Saddam Hussein and Hitler from which we can plan a successful plan of action. Thus predictions of exact repetitions are inherently flawed. But careful scrutiny of the validity of knowledge gained by our predecessors can provide us with a basis for future learning and investigation. Medical science is a good example, for when properly applied and validated, it will lead us to a brighter future. Predicting the exact form this future will take, however, is highly tenuous.

Exemplifying the wild inaccuracy of some predictions is wonderfully detailed in the entertaining passage quoted below that describes what many had predicted would happen as the clock struck midnight on Dec 31, 1999 heralding the onset of a new millennium: I quote portions of this colorful article by Denis Dutton from New Zealand, published in 2009 in the New York Times looking back at this presumably "momentous" event:

"There was a particular unease in the air. The so-called Y2K problem, the inability of computers to read dates beyond 1999, threatened to turn Jan. 1, 2000 into a nightmare. As the turn of the century loomed, it seemed that humankind faced a litany of horrors. Haywire navigation controls might cause aircraft to fall from the skies. Electricity grids, water systems and telephone networks would be knocked out, while nuclear power plants would be subject to meltdown. Savings and pension accounts would be wiped out in a general bank failure. A cascade of breakdowns in communication and commerce would create vast shortages of food and medicine, which would, in turn, produce riots, lawlessness and social collapse. Even worse, ICBMs might rise from their silos unbidden, spreading death across the globe. Problems were going to affect millions of tiny computer chips found everywhere. Elevators would die, G.P.S. devices would stop working and dishwashers would dry the food onto the plates before trying to

rinse it off. Even ordinary cars might spontaneously accelerate to fatal, uncontrollable speeds, with brakes failing to respond. The Rev. Jerry Falwell suggested that Y2K would be the confirmation of Christian prophecy, 'God's instrument to shake this nation, to humble this nation.' The Y2K crisis might incite a worldwide revival that would lead to 'the rapture of the church.' Along with many survivalists, Mr. Falwell advised stocking up on food and guns.

As clocks hit midnight on Dec. 31, 1999, Champagne and skyrockets were the only explosions of interest, since telephones, ATMs, cars, computers and airplanes worked just fine in New Zealand. We waited for news of the calamities sure to hit countries that had ignored Y2K. However, exactly 10 years ago today, as the date change moved on through the Far East, India, Russia, the Middle East and Europe, it became apparent that it made little difference whether you lived in Britain, which at great expense had revamped many of its computer systems, or the lackadaisical Ukraine, which had ignored the issue. In the United States, the Small Business Administration calculated that 1.5 million businesses had undertaken no Y2K remediation. On Jan. 3, it received about 40 phone calls from businesses that had experienced minor faults, like cash registers that misread the year "2000" as "1900" (which seemed everywhere the single most common error caused by Y2K). Knowing our computers is difficult enough. Harder still is to know ourselves, including our inner demons. From today's perspective, the Y2K fiasco seems to be less about technology than about a morbid fascination with end-of-the-world scenarios."

The passage above is self-explanatory. We can only emphasize the serious errors that can emanate from application of intuitive or apparently "rational" principles to predict the future. Even though, in retrospect, this whole issue seemed quite silly, we must attempt to free ourselves from our own hindsight bias.

THE ILLUSION OF VALIDITY

Experts in many fields who attempt to predict future events are usually wrong. But despite this, such individuals continue to emanate an aura of invincibility. This is called *the illusion of validity*. What seems to be the common attribute of these so-called pundits is the certainty and logic with which they deliver their well-crafted messages. They often appear on television and may command large followings. Yet, when subjected to objective analysis, they often produce predictions or other "truths" that are downright false. Moreover, even when proven inaccurate, they are able to ignore the actual facts and behave as if nothing had actually disproved their beliefs.[40] Their ability to convince others of their beliefs presents the major challenge—and danger—to society in general. Why people succumb to this illusion of validity is complex, and probably composed of a mixture of biases rooted in the eagerness with which we are willing to accept, without questioning, superficial conclusions, which may be reinforced by the influence of other believers.

Perhaps the quintessential example of the illusion of validity throughout all history was that of Adolf Hitler. Through highly developed and forceful oratorical skills, he presented apparently "logical" beliefs that his race and country were superior to all others. He often relied on bogus pseudoscientific information as "proof" of their racial superiority and that they were destined to rule the world. Needless to say, so compelling were his messages he succeeded in leading huge numbers of his own people, as well as countless others, to their deaths. Hitler's enormous crimes were facilitated by the willingness of his masses to believe his forceful and false "logic." Obviously, had his public been highly skeptical of such nonsense, the world would have been saved from unspeakable horror. Although far more extreme, is this

---

[40] Kahneman D. Thinking, Fast and Slow. Farrar, Straus and Giroux, New York, 2011, pp. 209-220.

disingenuousness really different from that demonstrated by many leaders—political and otherwise—throughout the world today, including the U.S.A? At least in this country, skepticism is imbedded in the fabric of our constitution, guaranteeing freedom of speech that does not allow for the suppression of healthy disbelief.

SECTION TWO: HEALTH FALLACIES AND MISCONCEPTIONS

⌇⌇ *Chapter Eleven* ⌇⌇

THE PLACEBO AND ITS EFFECTS

"The art of medicine consists of amusing the patient while Nature cures the disease"

Voltaire

A placebo is defined as "an inert medication used for its psychological effect, or for purposes of comparison in an experiment." This generally applies to the customary performance of a controlled, double-blind study to determine the efficacy of a new treatment. But a placebo also includes any treatment that exerts no physical effect on a disease. These "treatments" are often discovered to be ineffective months or even years after administration, and can include virtually any type of intervention—such as simple encounters with medical professionals, physical manipulations, and even surgical procedures.

The *placebo effect* can thus be defined as any improvement in subjective discomfort or illness not explained by the effect of the treatment given. I have deliberately broadened the definition to include unconventional care providers such as faith healers and, for the most part, practitioners of alternative medicine. This effect also plays an important role in the daily practice of medicine for almost all mainstream medical caregivers.

Few people outside of the medical profession understand the power of the placebo effect. It has been aptly characterized as "something to control in clinical research, something to cultivate in clinical practice, and something present in all healing encounters."[41] Although not well understood, the mechanism of the placebo effect relates to the power of the mind to affect bodily sensations and functions. It is especially effective in relieving pain, anxiety, fatigue, insomnia, and depression, but can go far beyond these even to enhance the effectiveness of medical interventions with acknowledged physical benefit. With this expanded definition we can proceed to review some of the vast experience with this phenomenon, and lessons learned, over the past half century.

Based on a review of medical studies, placebos improve or relieve symptoms in a widely divergent percentage of individuals suffering from numerous medical conditions. But the cause for such variable responses depends on the type of illness treated, the context of its administration, and how long the subjects are observed.[42] For instance, when used to evaluate new drugs, researchers focus solely on the difference between the active drug and the placebo, and so the placebo effect itself is rarely analyzed or compared with an absence of treatment. Compared in this latter way, one study reported little difference between a placebo and no treatment;[43] however, this information is tempered by the inclusion of numerous physical diseases and did not evaluate the nature of the interaction between caregiver and patient. Pain, however, did show a significant placebo response when compared with no treatment.

Generally, symptoms unrelated to serious underlying organic diseases, such as pain or fatigue, are most likely relieved

---

[41] Thompson JJ, Ritenbaugh C, and Nichter M., *Reconsidering the Placebo Response from a Broad Anthropological Perspective.* Cult Med Psychiatry. 2009;33: 112–152.

[42] Benedetti F. *Placebo Effects. Understanding the mechanisms in health and disease.* Oxford University Press., New York, N.Y. (2009).

[43] Hróbjartsson A.and Gøtzsche PC N Engl J Med 2001; 344:1594-1602. Is the Placebo Powerless? — An Analysis of Clinical Trials Comparing Placebo with No Treatment.

by a placebo. That is not to say, however, that these symptoms are not real or are imagined. I believe the relief of symptoms in this context is real, but the underlying physiological mechanisms are not well understood. A beneficial response occurs most often when the treatment is provided by a caregiver who explains that s/he expects improvement. It is also most likely to occur in individuals who are, in general, highly receptive to suggestion.[44] Additionally, the responses are more profound when a given medication is thought to be more expensive than a cheaper one.[45]

Perhaps the most potent placebo effects result from physical interventions, such as acupuncture. Recent studies have shown marked improvement with either traditional acupuncture, or a sham which employs superficial needling at non-acupuncture points. For example, in a trial of over 1,100 patients with chronic low back pain who received ten 30-minute sessions over five weeks,[46] the improvement rate after six months was 48% for traditional acupuncture and essentially the same for the sham procedure, compared to 27% for patients receiving customary care (physiotherapy plus as-needed pain medication), clearly confirming the placebo effect. The same observations have been found with migraine and tension-type (formerly called tension) headaches, irritable bowel syndrome, chronic low back pain, and even arthritis of the knee.

These findings establish two important points; the sham procedure is as effective as the real procedure, qualifying both as effective placebos, and the efficacy of both acupuncture

---

[44] De Pascalis V., Chiaradia C and Carotenuto E. *The contribution of suggestibility and expection to placebo analgesia phenomenon in an experimental setting.* Pain. 2002; 96; 393-402.
[45] Waber RL. Shiv B, Carmon Z, and Ariely D. *Commercial features of placebo and therapeutic efficacy.* JAMA 2008;299:1016-7.
[46] Haake M, Muller HH, Schade-Brittinger C, et al. *German Acupuncture Trials (GERAC) for chronic low back pain: randomized, multicenter, blinded, parallel-group trial with 3 groups.* Arch Intern Med. 2007;167:1892–1898.

procedures far exceeded those of ordinary medical management, indicating that the placebo effect is powerful indeed. Moreover, it demonstrates that acupuncture is likely only effective as a placebo. These and many other similar trials strongly suggest that this type of invasive but safe intervention, characterized by an elaborate treatment ritual and frequent clinician-patient interaction, may be a potent method of interpersonal healing by means of the placebo effect.[47] In general, physical manipulations demonstrate a more profound beneficial effect than do placebo tablets, as will be discussed further regarding chiropractic treatment.

A recent study[48] involving patients suffering from irritable bowel disorder reinforces the importance of personal interaction in any treatment encounter. In this study, patients received sham acupuncture twice a week for three weeks. In one (first) group, initial communication between practitioner and patient was businesslike and limited to 5 minutes; in the second, there was a forty-five-minute conversation with the practitioner at the initial visit regarding the patient's condition. This talk was purposefully supportive, with the idea of promoting positive expectations of acupuncture therapy. A third group received no treatment. Patients in the second group had superior outcomes of symptom relief and quality of life compared to those in the first group, which in turn had better outcomes than those in a third group who received no treatment. At three weeks after the "treatment," 62% of patients in the second group reported adequate symptom relief, compared with 44% in the first group and 28% in the third group.

This experiment suggests that simulation of treatment can account for therapeutic benefit. When enhanced by supportive

[47] Kaptchuk TJ. *The placebo effect in alternative medicine: Can the performance of a healing ritual have clinical significance?* Annals of Internal Medicine. 2002;136(11):817–825.

[48] Kaptchuk TJ, Kelley JM, Conboy Tversky A and Kahneman D. Judgment under Uncertainty: Heuristics and Biases Science, New Series, Vol. 185 (1974), pp. 1124-1131 and Arch Intern Med. 2008; 168(15): 1629–1637.

communication, however, the placebo response is dramatic. Thus, the placebo effect is closely bound to interpersonal contact.

Recognizing that the placebo effect is so closely bound to interpersonal contact, Kleinman et al.[49] advocate an informal process of medical psychotherapy as a basic component of care, focusing on the experience of chronically ill patients: "It is of the utmost importance that physicians achieve the highest possible placebo effect rates. To do this, doctors must establish relationships that resonate empathy and genuine concern for the well-being of their patients." They add that "The chief sources of therapeutic efficacy are the development of a successful therapeutic relationship and the rhetorical use of the practitioner's personality and communicative skills to empower the patient and persuade him toward more successful coping."

Sham surgeries have also demonstrated dramatic placebo effects. As mentioned earlier (Chapter Two), there was, in the 1950s, a common belief that individuals suffering from angina pectoris (chest pain originating from the heart) could benefit from the surgical ligation (closure) of the internal mammary arteries. Because of the tenuous nature of this hypothesis, a group of researchers divided eighteen volunteer individuals into two groups. Half received the ligation procedure, and the others received only superficial incisions on chest without ligation.[50] None of the participants was aware of which treatment s/he received. Surprisingly, both groups experienced marked, equal improvement in their symptoms. Of the entire group, fifteen experienced total relief of their symptoms after the procedures, and this relief persisted for periods up to one year. Very shortly after this study

---

[49]Kleinman A, Guess HA and Wilendtz IS. (2002). An overview. In: HA Guess et. al. *The Science of the Placebo Effect: Toward an Interdisciplinary Research Agenda.* pp. 1-32. BMJ Books, London.
[50] Dimond EG, Kittle CF, and Crockett JE., *Comparison of internal mammary artery ligation and sham operation for angina pectoris,* Am. Journal of Cardiology, 5;1960: p. 483-486.

was published in 1960, this procedure was discredited and abandoned, but the experience added strong support to the concept that the placebo effect was indeed powerful.

The interaction between mind and body is so potent that it can affect the course and outcome of certain *organic*, or physical, diseases. Mental depression is a well-known cause of poor outcomes in patients who have suffered myocardial infarctions. The cause of this relationship is not well understood. In those who suffered an attack, treatment with antidepressant drugs has been found to improve not only quality of life but also probably reduces recurrent heart attacks and even mortality, although the data are currently too limited to enable a firm conclusion.[51] Since depression responds profoundly to placebos,[52] one questions whether the placebo effect could be lifesaving.

The placebo effect may be beneficial in physical conditions as Parkinson's disease,[53] asthma,[54] and duodenal ulcer and inflammatory gastrointestinal conditions.[55] Although placebos have no effect on progression of cancer, they have been found to

---

[51] Glassman A, O'Connor C, Califf R, et al. *Sertraline treatment of major depression in patients with acute MI or unstable angina.* J.A.M.A.288;701. 2002.

[52] Walsh BT, Seidman SN, Sysko R and Gould M. *Placebo response in studies of major depression: variable, substantial, and growing.* Journal of the American Medical Association. 2002; 287:1840-1847.

[53] Shetty N., Friedman JH, Kieburtz K, et al. *The placebo response in Parkinson's Disease. Parkinson Study* Group. Clinical Neuropharmacology, 1999; 22:207-212.

[54] Luparello TJ, Lyons HA, Bleeker ER and McFadden ER. *Influence of suggestion on airways reactivity in asthmatic subjects,* Psychosomatic Medicine. 1968;30:819-825.

[55] Musial F, Klosterhalfen S and Enck P. *Placebo responses in patients with gastrointestinal disorders.* World Journal of Gastroenterology, 2007; 13:3425-3429..

reduce associated symptoms of pain, loss of appetite, anxiety, and depression.[56]

As one might anticipate, the placebo effect influences *erectile dysfunction* (ED). In a large analysis of Viagra versus placebo, Viagra was 57% effective in promoting successful sexual intercourse and a placebo resulted in a 21% success rate. One humorous response to these figures is a suggestion that men should try the placebo before using Viagra, for it could at least save money.

Of the manifold responses to the placebo, what is perhaps most amazing is its effect on physical sports performance. Enhancement of performance has been demonstrated in several trials. Clark et al[57] provided one notable example, when they studied the endurance of forty-three cyclists in a 40 kilometer timed trial. After suitable allocation into subgroups, those given placebos that were told they had received performance-enhancing carbohydrate performed 3.8% better than those given the same drink but told it was a placebo. Similar observations have been made in studies of muscle endurance and power in other athletes.[58] This raises the intriguing—albeit facetious—question: Should the administration of performance-enhancing placebos be considered "doping," and worthy of disqualification from competition?

The placebo effect clearly reflects the strong interplay between brain and body, and recipient and caregiver. More dramatic treatments, such as mechanical or surgical procedures, seem to evoke the greatest response. I believe that the personality

---

[56] Chvetzoff G. and Tannock IF. Placebo effects in oncology. *Journal of the National Cancer Institute. 2003; 95:19-29.*

[57] Clark VR. Hopkins WG, Hawley JA, and Burke LM. *Placebo effect of carbohydrate feeding during a 40-km cycling time trial.* Medical Sciences and Sports Exercise, 2000; 32:1642-1647.

[58] Beedie CJ, Coleman DA, and Foad AJ. *Positive and negative placebo effects resulting from the deceptive administration of an ergogenic aid.* International Journal of Sport, Nutrition, Exercise and Metabolism. 2007; 17:259-269.

of the caregiver strongly influences the results. Some physicians likely obtain optimum results by having a *placebo personality*—a positive and upbeat attitude toward an expected successful outcome. Additionally, of all patients seen in most general clinics, I would estimate that approximately 50%–70% have self-limiting conditions that will improve or resolve without treatment. This means any action taken by a physician will usually be followed by a favorable outcome and, according to the post hoc fallacy, both the patient and physician are seduced into believing the treatment brought about subsequent improvement. Thus, all practitioners, legitimate or otherwise, will achieve success through a combination of natural outcome, placebo effect and post-hoc reasoning. This can easily account for the apparent success of alternative medicine and faith healing.

The mechanism for the placebo's influence on brain/body connection had always been obscure until clues began to surface in the 1970s. The discovery of substances produced by the brain, called endorphins, has provided one possible answer to this enigma, at least in regard to the role of the placebo in combating pain. Endorphins are chemically similar to opiates like morphine and, therefore, likely provide pain relief. But does the placebo stimulate the brain's production of endorphins? The answer is they probably do, for one study demonstrated that Naloxone, a drug that blocks the physical effects of morphine, also was capable of nullifying relief of pain that was attributable to the placebo effect.[59] This may account for some of the real and physical pain relief afforded by placebos.

Since standard medical caregivers are keenly aware of the placebo effect, it is not surprising that this principle would be applied in clinical practice. Placebos may be administered in a "subtle" form, wherein a barely effective medication (such as a

---

[59] Levine JD, Gordon NC, Fields HL. The mechanism of placebo analgesia. Lancet. 1978; (8091):654-7.

mild tranquilizer) is given together with strong reassurance that said nostrum will be effective. Highly attenuated preparations are said to be "homeopathic" in nature, which is simply a form of alternative medicine (Chapter Thirteen). Vitamin B12, when given by injection in the absence of its deficiency, provides a more dramatic example of this effect (Chapter Fourteen). Probably less often, a medication without any physical effect whatever may be delivered with the same fanfare. Actual surveys of practitioners in mainstream medicine confirm the widespread use of placebos: in a study by Nitzan and Lichtenberg,[60] 60% of physicians and nurses used placebos, usually as often as once a month or more, and in most cases the patients were told they were receiving "real" medication. Of this latter group, 94% reported they found placebos generally effective. Another survey among academic physicians in the United States[61] disclosed that 45% had used placebos in clinical practice, most commonly to reduce anxiety and as supplemental treatment for physical problems. As many as 96% of these physicians believed placebos can have therapeutic effects, and 40% reported placebos could even benefit patients' physical problems. These studies serve to add additional support garnered worldwide from earlier surveys showing the same overall findings. Very few practitioners in any of these surveys considered placebo-giving as immoral or worthy of prohibition. Regardless of one's opinion about this issue, however, the placebo's safety profile is absolutely unbeatable.

PLACEBOS + HUCKSTERS = DEVILISH OUTCOMES

What happens when the hucksters with evil intentions tap into the power of the placebo effect? The early 20th century was

---

[60] Nitzan U and Lichtenberg P. *Questionaire survery on use of placebo*. British Medical Journal, 2004; 329:944-946.
[61] Sherman R. and Hickner J. *Academic physicians use placebos in clinical practice and believe in the mind-body connection*. Journal of General Internal Medicine, 2007; 23:7-10.

marked by many such shady characters, whose practices often produced painful, if not deadly, outcomes.

For example, Viagra and its ilk have helped satisfy aging men's near-universal desire to recapture their youthful sexual virility. This powerful yearning, present since antiquity, was the catalyst for one of the greatest scams of all time. When the desire for youthful vigor was combined with the placebo effect and the widespread gullibility of much of the population, there was an explosion of near-nuclear force.

John R. Brinkley (1885–1942)[62] was a faux doctor who, after failing to receive a legitimate medical degree, purchased a fake diploma from the Eclectic Medical University of Kansas City, Missouri, for $500. This gave him the right to practice medicine, without a formal examination, in Missouri, Arkansas, Kansas, and a few other states. In 1917, while serving as resident physician at a meatpacking company, he became interested in the vigorous mating activities of goats headed for slaughter. (Maybe the goats knew what fate lay ahead and wanted to make the most their time left.) After leaving this job, Brinkley established a private practice in Milford, Kansas. A local farmer came to see him, complaining of a sagging libido—now known as ED, or erectile dysfunction.

Brinkley, remembering the goats, told his patient that what he needed were some goat glands. The farmer allegedly responded by stating, "So, Doc, put 'em in. Transplant 'em." So Brinkley did just that, implanting a goat testicle into the patient's scrotum. This created the ideal scenario for a placebo effect—apparently supportive doctor-patient interaction and a dramatic surgical procedure. Predictably, the farmer returned within days to inform Brinkley that his libido was restored, and so began the saga. After several replications of this procedure, Brinkley's fame spread rapidly, resulting in an abundance of testimonials and lots of cash.

---

[62] Brock P. Charlatan: *America's Most Dangerous Huckster, the Man Who Pursued Him, and the Age of Flimflam.* Crown Publishers, New York. 2008.

He was charging $750 (approximately $6,500 in today's money) per transplant, yet couldn't keep up with the demand. Interestingly, Brinkley declared the procedure best suited to the intelligent and was inappropriate for the "stupid type." This psychological ploy meant that, provided you didn't consider yourself stupid, you had to admit that the operation was successful.

The proposed benefits of the procedure soon extended far beyond male virility. Brinkley claimed that it could cure twenty-seven ailments, including everything from dementia to emphysema to flatulence. His clientele included foreign dignitaries and even women. For a higher price, he transplanted human testicles obtained from convicts on death row (hopefully after they'd been executed).

Brinkley amassed a fortune, which enabled him to expand his empire. He dispensed phony medical advice over a radio station that he had purchased, usually coupled with prescriptions for useless or dangerous medications which were obtainable, of course, through one of his collaborating pharmacies. The prescriptions were sold at greatly inflated prices, from which Brinkley received generous kickbacks.

His domain eventually imploded under the pressure of the revocation of his medical license and the many lawsuits brought by patients and their families who had experienced infections and even death from his inept surgical procedures. He was also pressured relentlessly by the American Medical Association under the direction of Morris Fishbein, MD, the editor of its official journal (JAMA) and the medical equivalent of Eliot Ness.[§] In 1938, Fishbein published a two-part series called "Modern Medical Charlatans," which included a thorough repudiation of Brinkley's career, as well as the exposure of his questionable medical

---

[§] Eliot Ness became famous as the federal agent who led an incorruptible group of law enforcement officers dubbed "The Untouchables," the ones who brought down Chicago gangster Al Capone in the 1930s.

credentials. This was the final straw. After an unsuccessful lawsuit against Fishbein, Brinkley died penniless in 1942.

What lessons can we derive from this story? First, Brinkley's transplant procedures obviously provided no physical benefits. The implanted gonads, devoid of blood supply and inevitably rejected as foreign tissue—would have rapidly disintegrated. The minute amounts of testosterone contained in the implanted gonads would also have rapidly disappeared, and there is little evidence that this hormone would have been beneficial. Even purified and given in large amounts, its use for male impotence is problematic, except for the unusual individual who is truly testosterone deficient (Chapter Eighteen).

So, how can we explain the claimed successes of Brinkley's transplants? The major benefit would likely have stemmed from the placebo effect, enhanced by the high cost. The apparent benefits were likely supported by the need of the victims to avoid the embarrassment of admitting that they were stupid enough to have consented to a bogus procedure.

Brinkley's clever exploitation of the media provides another compelling lesson. The willingness of the public to pay high prices for useless remedies in response to this type of marketing hype confirms the presence and enormous power of the placebo effect and presages the successful exploitation of today's media.

The Brinkley saga demonstrates that, as long as sizeable portions of the populace are sufficiently credulous, the groundwork is present for unscrupulous healers of all types. Like the Hydra of Greek mythology, a multi-headed beast whose severed heads regenerated, snake oil continues to be resurrected. However, thanks to professional credentialing organizations and governmental watchdog agencies, Brinkley's blatant hucksterism is unlikely to recur now or in the future. Nevertheless, charlatans continue to operate most commonly in the safe havens afforded by various alternative medical fields.

THE "REVERSE" PLACEBO EFFECT": THE BRAIN AS A CAUSE OF ILLNESS

As presented above, the brain can be a powerful cause of relief—or even cure—of many illnesses. This effect is based, at least in part, on the positive anticipations from placebo treatments. But the flip side of this coin, illness resulting from expectation or fear of a bad effect, can be even more powerful. This has been labeled the "*nocebo*" effect, or the "placebo's evil twin"[63]   A nocebo response refers to harmful, unpleasant, or undesirable effects a subject manifests after receiving a placebo. These reactions are due basically to a subject's pessimistic belief and expectation that the inert drug will produce negative consequences. The actual responses range widely in nature, often taking the form of headaches, gastrointestinal upset, and many others. If the administration is accompanied by warnings of specific potential reactions, those effects are more apt to actually materialize. This fact alone accounts for why almost all drug trials demonstrate rates of undesirable "side effects" in the control (placebo) group. This provides ample reason for why proper research must include these latter comparisons.

But negative or fearful expectations extend beyond placebo effects. During my training in medical school, I learned about symptoms of many "dread diseases," frightening me into thinking that I may be developing each successive disease. As a result, I could actually "feel" a wide variety of symptoms shortly after reading their descriptions. Most of my fellow students also reluctantly admitted to similar experiences. Only after repeated exposures to these awful diseases did we become desensitized and were no longer subject to these unpleasant fears and bodily

---

[63] Reid B. Washington Post, April 30, 2002; Page HE01.

sensations. Another example with which we are all familiar is that of motion sickness. This clearly physical discomfort is common to many, often affecting those riding in the back of a bumpy automobile. But, curiously, those doing the driving or sitting in the front row are far less afflicted, clearly a result of brain function— brought about, to some extent, by a differing focus of attention. These are the simple demonstrations of how the mind can influence our physical sensations. But beyond these types of examples, the matter becomes much more complex.

Several common maladies seem to emanate solely from the brain, often called "psychosomatic" or "somatoform" disorders. These usually feature various aches and pains not explainable by objective medical testing. I believe these symptoms are really felt, i.e., they are not "all in the head," as is sometimes alleged. By contrast, pure fakery of symptoms, i.e. malingering, falls outside of this discussion. Sometimes these disorders are hidden behind other names such as psychogenic arthritis, fibromyalgia, and chronic widespread pain disorder. More focused areas of pain also can result from emotional factors, and these include, among others, tension-type headaches, back and chest pain. All are associated with emotional tension and/or depression, which often is associated with an unexplained sense of fear. These conditions are quite prevalent and can be severely disabling, persistent, and often resistant to treatment. Aggravating the anxiety imbedded in these conditions are occasional "panic attacks," which are marked by as extreme fear, sweating, breathlessness, light-headed sensations, numbness and tingling of the extremities, bodily pains (often in the chest), general weakness and even fainting. Extreme fear also usually triggers inappropriately rapid breathing—termed "hyperventilation"—which reduces carbon dioxide in the blood and contributes to many of the symptoms, including numbness and tingling of the extremities, weakness, and disturbed consciousness with fainting. Excessive breathing probably owes its existence to our evolutionarily adapted ancestors, whose anxious response in preparing for "flight or fight" triggering rapid breathing necessary to meet the upcoming heavy metabolic demands required by these activities. In modern times, however, anxiety and hyperventilation are not followed by increased physical activity and are thus inappropriate. This part of the disorder is easily combated by simply preventing the loss of carbon dioxide by either breath holding or rebreathing air in a simple paper bag. These maneuvers not only relieve these symptoms but help to allay the underlying fear and anxiety that initially triggered the attack. This combination of emotionally induced symptoms combined with the real physical consequences of hyperventilation is quite common, and may account for as much as ten percent of individuals seen in general medical clinics.

High blood pressure represents a physical disease often believed to have a mental component derived from the stresses and strains of everyday living. The complex nature of this disorder is evident, however, by the fact that efforts to treat emotional tension alone are seldom effective for its treatment.

Additional illnesses originally thought to have a primary psychological cause are now believed more complex. For instance, peptic ulcer was once thought of as being purely caused by stress, but later research revealed that that a bacterium (*Helicobacter pylori)* caused 80% of ulcers. Nevertheless, four out of five people harboring this potentially infectious agent do not develop ulcers. Thus an expert panel convened by the Academy of Behavioral Medicine Research concluded that ulcers are not merely a bacterial disease and that mental factors do indeed play a significant role.

Some disorders defy classification as purely physical, mixed psychosomatic, or completely somatoform. For instance, irritable colon (bowel) disorder was once considered as having purely mental causes, but subsequent research has shown significant differences in the behavior of the intestines in these sufferers. On the other hand, there are no actual structural changes in these individuals and research shows that stress and emotions are still aggravating factors in producing the unpleasant symptoms of this disorder.

Inasmuch as almost all physical illnesses have associated mental factors that determine their onset, presentation, clinical course, and susceptibility to treatment, there is little benefit in classifying disorders as purely physical or mixed psychosomatic. All management strategies must include identification of stress and include its remediation whenever possible.

A fascinating disorder with purely mental origins is called "sociogenic illness," or less commonly "mass hysteria," or "conversion disorder," a condition that usually occurs in several individuals within a group, but has no identifiable physical cause. It demonstrates how suggestion can produce apparently physical ailments, which can be quite variable, including blindness, nausea, headache, paralysis, inability to speak, and many others. One recent example (January, 2012) was that of fifteen teenage girls in upstate New York who reported a mysterious outbreak of spasms, tics, and "seizures." Although the initial trigger in this particular instance was unknown, most of these outbreaks result from stress to one individual that rapidly spreads by unconscious mimicry. This disorder has a predilection for young girls, but may involve other groups. Additional examples are too numerous to list, but a few notable examples follow: In the fall of 2007, approximately eight girls at a Roanoke, Va. high school developed strange-twitching symptoms similar those mentioned above. After spending $30,000 in the search, investigators found no environmental cause. Earlier in 2007, a mysterious illness swept through a Catholic boarding school in Chalco Mexico, causing six-hundred girls to suffer fever, nausea and buckling knees that left many unable to walk. Batteries of tests revealed no physical explanation.

Finally, another bizarre incident of probable sociogenic illness involved a cancer patient, Gloria Ramirez, in California. In 1994 Ramirez, suffering from terminal cancer and experiencing chest pain and stomach upset, was brought into the local Hospital's emergency department by paramedics. After drawing blood from the patient, several members of the hospital staff noted an ammonia-like smell and began to faint. Other members of the staff attended to their fallen comrades and attempted to treat Ramirez, who died shortly thereafter. The emergency department was evacuated, and a thorough search for a toxin revealed nothing. A State study of the incident concluded that Mass Sociogenic Illness was the cause. Although they definitely could not rule out the possibility that some workers were exposed to some type of unidentified poisonous substance, this remains doubtful. Although these cases, and many others, remain mysteries, and a toxin/poison usually can never be completely excluded, the large number of such similar instances lends support to the enormous power of suggestion and mimicry in producing real physical symptoms

❧ *Chapter Twelve* ❧

FAITH HEALING

"In GOD we trust, all others bring data."

Robert L. Fischer

A ccording to the dictionary, *faith healing* is the belief that religious faith can bring about healing—either through prayers or rituals that, according to adherents, evoke a divine presence and power toward correcting disease or disability. It can involve prayer, a visit to a shrine, or simply a strong belief in a supreme being. Although found in many religions, it is perhaps best known in connection with Christianity and the New Testament. *Spiritual healing*, however, makes no attempt to seek divine intervention, relying more on alternative medicine, sometimes combined with a distrust of or lack of confidence in standard medical care.

The placebo effect allows faith healing to gain traction in the general community, especially when reinforced by the dynamic personalities of religious leaders or cultists who perform the *laying on of hands.* This provides the important physical element noted in conjunction with the placebo effect. The physical contact between the healer and the sufferer in a group setting provides a powerful psychological incentive for the latter to show an immediate salutary response. The need to acknowledge immediate improvement or cure is further supported by the social pressure to avoid the embarrassment that would accompany the denial of any response. Of course, audiences cannot fail to be impressed by such dramatic responses, a factor that likely entices future recruits.

Although many such leaders are undoubtedly sincerely motivated to aid the sick and disabled, the elements of financial greed and fame are frequently inextricably associated. Stemming from obvious desperation, individuals suffering from the most severe and dread diseases such as cancer, are especially vulnerable to the superficial appeal of such claims. According to the American Cancer Society (ACS), although a small percentage of people with cancer have been known to experience remissions unexplained by the scientific community, "available scientific evidence does not support claims that faith healing can actually cure physical ailments. Death, disability, and other unwanted outcomes have occurred when faith healing was elected instead of medical care for serious injuries or illnesses."

The best and most accurate analysis of faith healing I have encountered can be found in William Nolen's book, titled "Healing: A Doctor in Search of a Miracle."[64] Dr. Nolen, a busy surgeon, expended enormous time and effort to detect evidence of physical healing that was accomplished by faith healers, religious or otherwise. His effort offers a rare and objective vignette into an obscure world.

Surprisingly, Nolen approaches the subject with an open mind, and goes to great lengths to interview several such healers, observe the procedures, and follow up on the results with recipients when possible. He concluded that such healers were either charlatans or religious zealots believing they were endowed with supernatural powers. The degree to which monetary reward influenced their ministrations was beyond the scope of his investigation, but it must have been significant. From the preceding discussion of the placebo, the reader can anticipate his findings.

First, he notes that in the case of organic diseases, such as cancer, multiple sclerosis, deforming arthritis, strokes, and other forms of paralysis, there is no evidence that any cures have ever occurred. All of us in medical practice are aware of an occasional,

---

[64] Nolen WA, *Healing: A doctor in Search of a Miracle*, Fawcett Crest, New York, N.Y., 1974.

but rare, case of cancer that goes into spontaneous remission or even disappears totally in the absence of treatment, but Nolen was unable to document any such examples that could have been attributed to healers. Conversely, he encountered many cases of *functional*, or psychosomatic, conditions that did show improvement, including tension-type or migraine headaches, irritable colon syndrome, back pain without of physical deformity, and others. These examples would be amenable to standard medical care, especially in an understanding and caring environment. Unfortunately, most physicians have inadequate time or inclination to devote adequate resources to these types of problems.

Finally, Nolen discusses conditions that have both physical and functional components, such as some forms of arthritis, duodenal ulcer disease, and high blood pressure, among others. In these examples, associated pains, subjective weakness, and anxiety can be markedly alleviated by the power of suggestion alone, abetted by an intensive interview with the caregiver, and supplemented further by the administration of a medication. All this likely represents the placebo effect.

To quote Dr. Nolen: "What we doctors must do is to explain all this to our patients. Tell them that we are not miracle men or women—that nature does a lot more to heal the sick than we do—that, in effect, much of the time patients heal themselves. In the past we've been too busy to tell patients all they have a right to know about their diseases and about healing in general. We've rationalized our point of view by saying 'without a medical education it's too difficult to understand.' And because we've left patients in the dark, they've gone off to healers. In the future we must share our knowledge with our patients." His statement remains largely true today; however, because of increasing time and financial constraints, physicians are, in general, still unable to devote adequate time to this type of patient education. Unfortunately, those who would benefit most from intensive investments of time are usually those with non-life-threatening functional disorders. It is logical for most physicians to prioritize their time in the effort to administer the most care to those having serious and life-threatening physical disorders.

Despite the fact that most patients are now better able to supplement information about their ailments from the Internet, I believe that those suffering from functional illnesses will continue to seek sources outside mainstream medicine for care and attention. It is equally inevitable and understandable that many who suffer from cancer and other deadly conditions will also seek unconventional avenues out of desperation, grasping at any possibility after having been told that conventional medicine has nothing further to offer. Rather than wasting money on worthless remedies, we would fare better channeling these funds into organizations devoted to fighting these diseases at a societal level, such as the American Cancer Society.

⟢ *Chapter Thirteen* ⟣

ALTERNATIVE MEDICINE

"From powerful causes spring the empiric's gains,
Man's love of life, his weakness, and his pains;
These first induce him the vile trash to try,
Then lend his name, that other men may buy."

George Crabbe

Alternative medicine may be defined as any healing practice that does not fall within the realm of conventional medicine. It is based on historical or cultural traditions, rather than on scientific evidence, and it has features resembling faith or spiritual healing. This definition includes a broad array of therapeutic interventions unstudied by conventional contemporary methods, and so it operates apart from evidence based medicine.

More than one-hundred-million Americans consume vitamins, minerals, herbal ingredients, amino acids, and other naturally occurring products in the form of dietary supplements. Of the huge number of unproven remedies on which over $28 billion yearly are spent, most are obtainable without a prescription from health food stores, many pharmacies, and through the internet. Most fall into the category of "herbal" medicines. In the present era, nearly one in five adults in the United States reports taking an "herbal" product.[65] For more than 5,000 years this was the only form of medicine. Even as recently as 1890, 59% of the listings in the US Pharmacopeia were herbal in origin. An herb can be any form of plant or plant product, including leaves, stems, flowers, roots and seeds. They are sold either raw or as extracts. The

---

[65]Bent S. *Herbal Medicine in the United States: Review of Efficacy, Safety, and Regulation.* J. Gen Intern Med. 2008; 23: 854–859.

resulting products usually contain multiple substances of various chemical types. Since any given herb contains several ingredients, some manufacturers try to create standardized herbal products by identifying a suspected active ingredient and altering the manufacturing process to obtain a consistent amount of this chemical, but such attempts themselves are fraught with considerable uncertainty created by variations in the analytical methods. For most herbs, the exact chemical, or combination of chemicals, that produces a biological effect is unknown, and it is therefore difficult—if not impossible—to create a precise "chemical fingerprint" of the optimum herbal product.

As one might anticipate, regulation of herbal products is a daunting challenge. The Dietary Supplement Health and Education Act (DSHEA) of 1994 classified herbs loosely as "dietary supplements," that is, "anything" that supplements the diet—a nebulous concept indeed. Supplements, therefore, may include vitamins, minerals, herbs, amino acids, enzymes, organ tissues, metabolites, extracts, or concentrates.

All ingredients sold in the U.S. before 1994 are allowed to be marketed without any evidence of efficacy or safety. Given the complexity of most ingredients and their combinations, accurate studies of safety are almost totally lacking. The Federal Act of 1994 (DSHEA) attempted to provide more regulation of the safety of these products, stipulating that ingredients introduced after that time must be accompanied by evidence that there is a "reasonable expectation of safety" (whatever that means) acceptable to the FDA. Unfortunately even this meager expectation has never been adequately enforced. The FDA has received notification of only 170 new supplement ingredients since 1994, despite an estimated 51,000 new supplements appearing on the market.[66]

---

[66] Cohen PA. *Assessing supplement safety—the FDA's Controversial Proposal.* New Eng. J. Medicine. 2012; 366; 389-391.

Because of these obvious shortcomings, the FDA proposed in July 2011 guidance clarifying evidence necessary to assess the safety of ingredients introduced after 1994. This involved documented history of use, formulation and proposed daily dose, and duration of consumption relative to historical standards. If a new ingredient was marketed in doses exceeding those historically used, or if formulated or synthesized in a new manner, the FDA would require animal and/or historical documentation for safety. These apparently more stringent regulations remain seriously flawed, e.g., the FDA would not require studies in humans for ingredients lacking evidence of historical use. Even prior use is relevant only if one would have expected to detect adverse effects, which has seldom been accomplished in careful analysis. Even more damning, however, the new guidance would not mandate that all data—both favorable an unfavorable—be submitted to the FDA; a manufacturer could perform multiple studies and submit only the favorable data.

Thus even if these new guidelines were enacted into law, they would provide little assurance to the public that many of these products were actually safe. From this information, we can conclude that, unless compelling evidence (see below) indicates that any of these supplements are effective for any disorder—which is seldom the case—one should avoid all of them.

A major difference between a drug and a dietary supplement is that dietary supplements may not claim to "diagnose, cure, mitigate, treat, or prevent specific illnesses." Consequently, dietary supplement manufacturers can make only general "structure/function" claims, which are often vaguely worded assertions of health benefits such as "support the body's natural defenses," "promote heart health," "better circulation," "increased energy," "better joint health and mobility," etc. They regularly provide a disclaimer that their product "has not been evaluated by the Federal Drug Administration (FDA)." Their wording is regularly evasive, for claims to treat specific diseases cause products to be considered drugs. Firms making such assertions legally must follow FDA's premarket new drug approval process to show the products are safe and effective—an onerous and expensive task. Singh and Ernst,[67] have aptly summarized this situation with the statement, "Conventional medicine and alternative medicine both have the same ambition, namely to cure the sick, and yet one is tightly regulated and the other operates in the medical equivalent of the Wild West. This means that patients who venture towards alternative medicine are at risk of being exploited, losing their money and damaging their health."

Angell and Kassirer[68] best sum up the feeling of the scientific community toward alternative medicine: "It is time for the scientific community to stop giving alternative medicine a free ride. There cannot be two kinds of medicine—conventional and alternative. There is only medicine that has been adequately tested and medicine that has not, medicine that works and medicine that may or may not work. Once a treatment has been tested rigorously, it no longer matters whether it was considered alternative at the outset. If it is found to be reasonably safe and effective, it will be accepted. But assertions, speculation, and testimonials do not substitute for evidence. Alternative treatments should be subjected to scientific testing no less rigorous than that required for conventional treatments." The authors state further that alternative medicine also distinguishes itself by an ideology that largely ignores biologic mechanisms, often disparages modern science, and relies on what are purported to be ancient practices and natural remedies, which are seen as being simultaneously more potent and less toxic than conventional medicine. Thus herbs or mixtures of them are considered superior to active compounds isolated in the

---

[67] Singh S. and Ernst E. *Trick or Treatment: The undeniable facts about alternative medicine.* W.W. Norton Co. New York and London, 2008. p. 281.
[68] Angell M, Kassirer JP. *Alternative medicine—the risks of untested and unregulated remedies* The New England Journal of Medicine 1998; 339:839–41.

laboratory. Notwithstanding these statements, unorthodox healing methods continue to be fervently and widely promoted.

Although lacking original scientific validation, these alternative measures were not always worthless or ineffective; historically, an occasional therapeutic agent has been discovered accidentally and found to be effective after careful observation of multiple case responses. Quinine is a good example. This compound occurs naturally in the bark of the cinchona tree, was first found centuries ago by the Quechua Indians of South America and found to have therapeutic properties against malaria. Later the Jesuits brought cinchona to Europe. The active compound was subsequently refined and has been used for many years in treating malaria, and is still used on a limited basis today.

The discovery of the medicinal value of *Digitalis purpurea* (foxglove plant) by William Withering (1741–1799) constituted a great milestone in early scientific medicine.[69] After having been trained as a physician, Withering's interests turned to botany, leading him to publish extensively on the classification and description of plants of England. After hearing about the use of a polyherbal treatment for *dropsy*, now called congestive heart failure, he somehow deduced that foxglove (digitalis) was most likely the active ingredient in the mixture. Over the next nine years, he tried preparations of various parts of the digitalis plant in treating this disorder. He refined the leaf into a powder, established the proper dose, and documented signs of overdose. Without recognizing that the heart was the underlying culprit in dropsy, Withering carefully studied the effects of digitalis on 163 patients suffering from this disorder. His results, published in 1785, were nothing short of miraculous. He described the rapid loss of

---

[69] Peck TW, Wilkinson KD (1950). William Withering of Birmingham MD. FRS. FLS. Bristol: John Wright and Sons.

excessive body fluid, improvement in breathlessness and vitality, and the slowing of excessively rapid heart rates. These observations have been repeatedly observed in following centuries, and are clearly related to the successful treatment of heart failure. Many modern studies have shown that this drug enhances the strength of contraction of the heart muscle. For this reason, one of the active ingredients of foxglove, digoxin, continues to be used for heart failure today.

Plain old aspirin also dates back to antiquity. Hippocrates, the father of modern medicine, who lived sometime between 460 BC and 377 BC, recorded the use of powder made from the bark and leaves of the willow tree to aid headache, pain, and fever. In 1897, chemists working at Bayer created a synthetically altered version of this compound, acetylsalicylic acid, and trademarked the name Aspirin. Not only was the drug found effective for pain and fever, but recent scientific research has demonstrated that it reduces blood clotting, and can thus help to prevent and treat heart attacks and strokes (Chapter Six). One additional potential advantage to those taking regular aspirin is its demonstrated ability to reduce the long-term risk for cancer of the colon, esophagus, stomach, bile ducts and breast.[70,71] In general, however, because of aspirin's occasional side effects such as excessive bleeding, I do not recommend its use unless coupled with the intent of reducing cardiovascular risk. This rather complex issue is best resolved in conjunction with one's individual physician.

The boundaries between conventional and alternative medicine sometimes blur because much common practice is based on older methods that lack firm research. Furthermore, evidence-

---

[70] Chan AT, and Giovannucci EL. *Primary Prevention of Colorectal Cancer* Gastroenterology. 2010; 138: 2029–2043.

[71] Algra AM, Rothwell PM. Effects of regular aspirin on long-term cancer incidence and metastasis: a systematic comparison of evidence from observational studies versus randomized trials. Lancet Oncol. 2012 Mar 20. [Epub ahead of print]

based procedures do not cover all possible scenarios. For instance, all currently accepted drugs are labeled with specific indications for their use, but additional uses that are not covered are often found, which results in what is called "off-label" use.

Many conditions encountered in medical practice have not yet been adequately studied scientifically, but the need for medical management cannot await the outcome of controlled trials that could take months or years to complete. The diagnosis and management of prostate cancer provides an excellent example. It often advances slowly and may not be symptomatic or fatal for many years. Therefore, the efficacy of various treatments—or no treatment at all—cannot be fully evaluated for long periods of time. This even calls into question the use of a common blood test, *prostate specific antigen* (PSA). If an elevated level is detected, indicating the likely presence of early prostatic cancer, we are often uncertain how to proceed. An individual having this malignancy may succumb to other conditions before he suffers symptoms or disability from a very slowly progressing prostate cancer.

Sometimes alternative medicine is added to conventional approaches. Then it is defined as *complementary/alternative medicine* (CAM). According to Steven Novella, editor of the website Science-Based Medicine, "this expression is a political/ideological entity, not a scientific one. It is an artificial category created for the purpose of promoting a diverse set of dubious, untested, or fraudulent health practices. It is an excellent example of the (successful) use of language as a propaganda tool."[72] In a review by Barnes et. al.,[73] 62% of adults used some form of CAM during the previous twelve months, most often for

---

[72] http://www.sciencebasedmedicine.org/index.php/national-health-interview-survey-2007-cam-use-by-adults/.

[73] Barnes PM, Powell-Griner E, McFann K, and Nahin, RL. *Complementary and alternative medicine use among adults: United States, 2002.* Seminars in Integrative Medicine. 2004;2:54-71.

back pain, head or chest infections, neck pain, joint pain or stiffness, and anxiety or depression. Unfortunately, however, as one of my colleagues aptly stated, "Attempts to mix scientific medicine with alternative medicine make about as much sense as mixing physics with metaphysics."

If scientific investigation establishes the safety and effectiveness of an alternative medical procedure, it becomes part of mainstream medicine and is no longer alternative, and may then become widely adopted by conventional practitioners. Digitalis and quinine are good examples of this phenomenon. But despite these exceptions, the vast majority of alternative treatments are not scientifically validated. They are at best, useless, and at worst, dangerous.

Alternative medicine includes chiropractic treatment , herbalism, traditional Chinese medicine, ayurvedic medicine, meditation, yoga, biofeedback, hypnosis, homeopathy, acupuncture, and nutritional-based therapies, among others. Contrasting with alternative medicine, osteopathic medicine and podiatry are now integrated into conventional medicine in the United States. In other countries, however, notably the United Kingdom, osteopathy is not.

Homeopathy is a form of alternative medicine in which practitioners claim to treat patients using highly diluted preparations that are believed to cause healthy people to exhibit symptoms that are similar to those exhibited by the patient (again demonstrating false logic). The collective weight of scientific evidence has found homeopathy to be no more effective than a placebo.

The basic principle of homeopathy, known as the "law of similar," is "let like be cured by like." This was first stated by German physician Samuel Hahnemann in 1796. This method, while of some historical interest, is no longer in general use. In some instances, however, caregivers may resort to this principle to achieve improvement specifically through the placebo effect.

CHIROPRACTIC TREATMENT

"It is a little too convenient that while chiropractors believe the body has the innate ability to heal itself, that gift doesn't extend to the backbone. For many chiropractors, it takes God to heal the body, but chiropractic to heal the spine."

Source unknown

Chiropractic theory is the brainchild of Daniel David Palmer, a grocer, who in 1895 postulated that the underlying cause of 95% of all diseases was interference with the body's nerve supply due to *subluxated* vertebrae (displaced spinal bones). He stated that subluxations interfered with the body's expression of "Innate Intelligence"—the "Soul, Spirit, or Spark of Life" that controlled the healing process. He proposed to remedy most diseases by manipulating, or adjusting, these problem areas.

The definition of vertebral subluxation is, however, controversial. The accepted standard medical definition of this term refers to significant structural displacement that can be visualized by means of imaging techniques, such as x-rays. On the other hand, chiropractors often suggest that a poorly functioning segment of the spine, whether displaced or not, should be referred to as a subluxation, which leads to altered function of the nerves, which supposedly leads to neurologic, musculoskeletal, and visceral disorders. Despite these tenuous and somewhat bizarre-sounding concepts, chiropractic has become an important component of the US health care system, and the largest alternative medical profession.

Although the core chiropractic belief remains the concept that the correcting spinal abnormalities will cure numerous diseases, there is a division within the field in which one group, called the *straights*, are at odds with the second group, the *mixers*.

Straights rely exclusively on spinal adjustments and adhere to the notion that subluxation "is the leading cause of disease in the world today."[74] Since the 1930s, straights have been in the minority; however, their status as purists and heirs of the lineage influences the profession disproportionately to their numbers. Mixers are more open to conventional medicine and mainstream scientific tenets. For today's mixers, subluxation is one of many causes of disease, which this translates into a greater use of therapies other than spinal manipulation.

Many chiropractors use conventional physical therapy techniques, such as corrective exercise, ice packs, bracing, bed rest, moist heat, and massage. Nutritional supplements are often added in mixer practice and, depending on state law, some chiropractors may provide acupuncture, homeopathy, herbal remedies, and even biofeedback. Despite these philosophical differences, adjusting the spine with the hands—the signature chiropractic gesture—is the unifying activity that allows chiropractic to create a coherent profession. Chiropractic manipulation is a method of moving vertebrae beyond the normal limit of motion, but not so far as to destroy the integrity of joint structure. The adjustment temporarily creates an increased range of motion. The patient feels the change and often hears a popping or cracking noise, which obviously adds a dramatic effect to the treatment.

Although they claim to relieve or cure of a wide range of diseases, chiropractic treatment the United States is usually directed at the widespread presence of pain, especially low back pain, neck pain, and headaches. Most authorities believe that about 69% of men and 88% of women develop tension-type headaches at some time during their lives. Such headaches can occur at any age, but most commonly begin during adolescence or young adulthood,

---

[74] Kaptchuk TJ. *The placebo effect in alternative medicine: Can the performance of a healing ritual have clinical significance?* Annals of Internal Medicine. 2002; 136(11):817–825.

with the highest frequency among those aged twenty to fifty years. They are often accompanied by neck pain. Estimations of the frequency of low back pain are equally impressive; between 70% and 80% of all adults experience low back pain at some point and, in any single year, more than 50% of Americans suffer from some type of low-grade back pain. Although most acute episodes resolve spontaneously, chronic pain is also common, and affects nearly a third of the American population.

Low back pain—both acute and chronic—is the scourge of most standard medical practitioners. In the majority of cases, standard x-rays show no clear abnormalities to explain the discomfort. Such pains are probably caused by muscle strain and spasm that may be produced or aggravated by emotional tension. Patients over forty often have minor degenerative changes of the vertebral column, but these rarely produce symptoms. These statistics open wide the door to alternative treatments. Of all patients seeking treatment from chiropractors, approximately 80% have musculoskeletal pains—at least 65% have back pain, but other symptoms may involve pain in the head, neck, and extremities.

Not surprisingly, many large surveys show that patients believe chiropractic works for them; most current and former chiropractic patients are likely satisfied with the treatment they received. Studies that compare patients' satisfaction with chiropractic versus conventional medicine in treating low back pain show a preference for chiropractic treatment.[75] The results of a recent survey of over 14,000 subscribers conducted by *Consumer Reports* echo those of other studies; 58% of respondents reported that chiropractic treatments "helped a lot." They also noted that spinal manipulation can be helpful for lower-back pain in the

---

[75] Kaptchuk TJ. *The placebo effect in alternative medicine: Can the performance of a healing ritual have clinical significance?* Annals of Internal Medicine. 2002;136(11):817.

short-term, but Consumers Union, the publisher of *Consumer Reports*, cautions that manipulations can aggravate structural problems, such as a herniated disk. For chronic back pain lasting more than twelve weeks, however, chiropractic did not appear to be better than general medical care, including physical therapy, exercises, and weight reduction.

But the back pain story doesn't end here. In recent years, surgical treatment for chronic back pain (defined as that persisting for three months to a year) has fallen into disrepute.[76] This is because active non-surgical management, consisting of rest, heat, massage, and analgesic medications, combined with a *cognitive-behavioral approach* (which supposedly identifies and modifies peoples' understanding of their pain and disability using cognitive restructuring techniques, such as imagery and attention diversion, or by modifying maladaptive thoughts, feelings, and beliefs) have been shown to provide just as much benefit as surgery for patients in whom there is no evidence of compression of spinal nerves.

These latter approaches resemble closely those of yoga,[77] another alternative therapy of questionable value, combining physical exercise, instruction in posture, and mental focus aimed at relaxation. Even in some patients who show evidence of compression of spinal nerves supplying other parts of the body, causing pain, numbness, or weakness in an arm or leg, conservative care can also be appropriate. If surgery, under many of these circumstances, is generally no better than the laying on of hands, one must logically suspect the placebo effect is largely responsible for much of this apparent benefit. Thus a caveat for anyone considering surgery—think twice or get a second medical opinion.

---

[76] Ibrahim T, Tleyjeh IM, and Gabbar O. *Surgical versus non-surgical treatment of chronic low back pain: a meta-analysis of randomized trials...* Int Orthop 2008; 32:107–113.

[77] Tilbrook HE et al. *Yoga for chronic low back pain.* Annals of Internal Medicine. 2011:155; 569-578.

So, how do we explain the apparent success of chiropractic treatment? There have been a few controlled studies, but most protocols were suboptimal and the results have been variable. In general, however, when compared with standard, rather passive methods such as heat, analgesics, and rest, chiropractic manipulation results in greater benefit in both acute and chronic back pain. Similar, less conclusive results have been found in individuals with neck pain and tension-type headaches. To my knowledge, chiropractic methods have not been compared to more active types of physical therapy such as massage, supervised exercise, and cognitive behavioral therapy. The results of such a study could be quite illuminating. In any event, there is no way to adequately assess the effect of lengthy personal contact and the laying on of hands that accompanies chiropractic treatment. The placebo effect may explain its apparent success, but the positive results in many patients cannot be denied.

Whether there is a proper place for chiropractic treatment in conventional medicine remains moot. Perhaps the most balanced account has been provided by Samuel Homola, D.C., a second-generation chiropractor who dedicated himself to defining the proper limits of chiropractic and to educating consumers and professionals about the field. In his 1963 book, *Bonesetting, Chiropractic, and Cultism,* he supported the appropriate use of spinal manipulation but renounced chiropractic dogma. His 1999 book, *Inside Chiropractic: A Patient's Guide,* provides an incisive look at chiropractic's history, benefits, and shortcomings. In his writings, Homola states, "The theory that a subluxation, or slight misalignment of a vertebra, can cause nerve interference that will affect organ function or general health is as implausible as the original 1895 theory. Chiropractors who subscribe to this theory manipulate the spine as a method of treatment for a host of organic conditions—an approach that has rightly been rejected by medical science. This is why the chiropractic profession has never received the full support of mainstream healthcare."

Generally, manipulation should be discontinued if symptoms worsen during the first week of treatment, or if no improvement occurs after two to four weeks. Since there is a total absence of evidence to suggest any benefit, it is never a good idea to continue ongoing manipulative treatment as maintenance therapy when symptoms are no longer present, especially in the case of neck manipulation, which entails some risk of potential damage to the spinal column.

To understand more fully the apparent success of chiropractic and other forms of alternative care, we must consider the type of individual most likely to benefit from them. As noted, large segments of the population suffer from chronic and recurrent musculoskeletal pains for which there is no physical explanation. These complaints are often accompanied by chronic fatigue and insomnia. Based on my experience, roughly 10%–20% of all patients fall into this category. An associated emotional component often accompanies these symptoms, meaning that the patients are anxious and may or may not be depressed as well. This psychological state promotes skeletal muscle tension, especially in the back, neck and head. It probably also lowers the *pain threshold*, meaning that pain experienced as normal by most individuals is disproportionately magnified by the sensitized mental state into seeming major. After testing to rule out physical disease, many physicians will stop, simply stating there is no or organic cause. They may state further that the underlying cause for the pain is emotional—that is, the pain is "all in your head." In response to this, most patients either conclude the doctor thinks the pain is not real, or worse, the patient is crazy and/or may need to see a psychiatrist. Even if the physician explains the problem in a more understanding and diplomatic fashion, many of these patients deny that the underlying emotional state could cause physical discomfort, believing instead that they are distraught or depressed because of the pains rather than the reverse.

Because of this thought reversal, the idea of accepting emotional support or psychiatric care is unacceptable. Further complicating the issue is the fact that many patients wish to have a physical explanation for their symptoms, something that has a name. Having such a diagnosis may serve several purposes. First, they can avoid the embarrassment of having a psychosomatic, or possibly imaginary, illness. Second, after they have been diagnosed with a presumably "organic" disease, they may get more sympathy and attention and control over family members and friends. Finally, having such a diagnosis may provide a ticket for limiting work at home or the office, and may even provide a basis for obtaining disability compensation.

Given these factors, such individuals often turn to alternative sources for care, particularly chiropractors. After x-raying the spine, the chiropractor may point out "abnormal shadows" that reveal the underlying source of their problem—subluxations. (I assure you that, after viewing a typical x-ray of the spine, I can point out something that looks a little odd, even if it's perfectly normal.) This can be accompanied by lengthy explanations, promoting further confidence in the caregiver. Most importantly, perhaps, is the laying on of hands to adjust the spine. This provides the ideal scenario for achieving the placebo effect. Additionally, any associated massage may relieve muscle spasms that contribute to the underlying pains.

The success of chiropractic care is easily explained by this combination of events. With such overall success, are these practitioners providing a real service to their patients? The answer to this question is yes—a qualified yes. The relief of symptoms is a plus, even though it usually results from a false premise, which is academically and morally troublesome. The result is also probably gained at an excessive cost to the system and patient. Also, potential harm could result from delaying standard medical care for those experiencing symptoms that could be caused by serious conditions, such as cancer. Moreover, additional risks include unnecessary exposure to x-rays, thus increasing slightly the long-term risk of developing all types of malignancies. Additional cautions include the slight risk of damage to the spinal column, especially the neck, which can result in serious neurologic consequences, including muscular paralysis and even death.

Readers, when considering chiropractic treatment, let the buyer beware.

THE POPULARITY OF ALTERNATIVE MEDICINE IN THE UNITED STATES

"Things will get better despite our efforts to improve them."

Will Rogers

Alternative medicine remains extremely popular.

The most common alternative therapies used in the United States in 2002 were prayer, 45.2%; herbalism, 18.9%; breath meditation, 11.6%; meditation, 7.6%; chiropractic treatment, 7.5%: yoga, 5.1%; body work, 5.0%; diet-based therapy, 3.5%; progressive relaxation, 3.0%; mega-vitamin therapy 2.8%; and visualization, 2.1%.

In 2004, a survey of nearly 1,400 US hospitals found that more than one in four offered alternative and complementary therapies such as acupuncture, homeopathy, and massage therapy.

A 2008 survey of US hospitals by Health Forum, a subsidiary of the American Hospital Association, found that more than 37% of responding hospitals indicated that they offer one or more alternative medicine therapies—up from 26.5% in 2005.

Additionally, hospitals in the southern Atlantic states were most likely to offer these methods, followed by the eastern and north-central states, then those in the middle Atlantic. More than 70% of these hospitals were in urban areas. The surveys conducted by the National Science Foundation also indicate the increasing popularity of alternative medicine.

What can we conclude from these statistics? Although there is no single answer, I believe these data reflect a combination of four factors: overutilization of standard medical facilities, which results in prolonged waits for treatment; limited time for in-depth interviews and explanations by caregivers; the placebo effect; and a post hoc effect—most illnesses are transient and will resolve spontaneously, meaning that any treatment will be viewed as curative. Because of these issues, I believe alternative medicine will remain popular for a long time.

Although seemingly counterintuitive, this trend benefits conventional medicine, to a degree, by its tendency to channel many individuals having non-lethal conditions away from already overburdened caregivers.

MORE ALTERNATIVE MEDICINE: A TALE OF TWO HOAXES

"Nothing more strikingly betrays the credulity of mankind than medicine. Quackery is a thing universal, and universally successful."

Henry David Thoreau

Although medical hoaxes abound throughout history, two examples provide insight into their dynamics and certain underlying common features. Notably, however, they have occurred recently, when society might have demonstrated greater enlightenment.

HOAX #1: CHELATION THERAPY

About thirty years ago, while I was attending an editorial board meeting of a national medical journal, several fellow board members complained that no one had critically challenged the practice of chelation therapy, which was widely promoted and gaining popularity around the country. Virtually the entire mainstream scientific medical community agreed this treatment fell outside standard methods, had never been critically tested, was almost certainly quackery, and was often used primarily for financial gain. Of course, anecdotal reports of successful outcomes were being spread by word of mouth, as well as being reported in the press.

This issue was then presented at our formal editorial board meeting, and when asked why scientific validation of such therapy had never been undertaken, the editor-in-chief responded that he was unable to find anyone interested in pursuing a project validating or refuting chelation therapy. After reflection, I realized this lack of interest was understandable. A properly conducted study would have required the enlistment of hundreds of volunteer subjects at multiple medical facilities, and would have required several years to complete. Since serious researchers are occupied with projects they consider important to advance medical science and treatment, these same individuals were not inclined to undertake a project that almost certainly was destined to invalidate a treatment already besmirched by many signs of shady practice.

So what is chelation therapy, and claims are made about it?[78] Well, the chelating agent is an organic chemical, ethylenediaminetetraacetic acid (EDTA), first synthesized in Germany in the 1930s. The word *chelate* refers to this chemical's ability to bind water-soluble heavy metals such as iron, mercury, lead, aluminum, and calcium. Through the chelation process,

---

[78] Atwood KC. Why the NIH Trial to Assess Chelation Therapy (TACT) Should Be Abandoned. Medscape J Med. 2008; 10: 115.

poisonous levels of toxic metals such as lead and mercury can be removed from the blood with lifesaving results.

After EDTA was found effective in removing toxic metals from the blood, some investigators postulated that arteriosclerotic arteries could be softened if the calcium in their walls was removed (another example of the intuitive fallacy). The first report of "successful" treatment came from Clarke et al., who reported in 1956 that patients having peripheral vascular disease caused by arteriosclerosis said they felt better after treatment with EDTA. Following that report, additional small studies showed beneficial results, but they did not use matched control patients, and so were not considered scientifically acceptable by today's standards.

In 1973, the American College for Advancement in Medicine (ACAM) was founded, and became the primary organization promoting chelation therapy. The group conducts courses, sponsors the *American Journal of Advancement in Medicine*, and administers a board certification program not recognized by the mainstream scientific community. ACAM's online directory lists about eight-hundred-fifty members; approximately five-hundred-fifty of those indicate that they practice chelation therapy.

In 1989, ACAM published a modified protocol for "the safe and effective administration of EDTA chelation therapy," calling for intravenous infusions including several B-vitamins and large doses of vitamin C. This solution is infused slowly over three-and-a-half to four hours, one to three times a week. The initial recommendation was a series of about thirty such treatments, with the possibility of more later, although candidates for this therapy were not specified. To their credit, however, lifestyle modifications were included in the program, including smoking cessation, exercise, and nutritional counseling. The number of treatments to achieve "optimal therapeutic benefit" for patients with symptomatic disease ran from twenty to forty, and up to one hundred or more over several years, because "full benefit does not normally occur for up to three months after a series is completed." Also, "follow-up treatments could be given once or twice monthly for long-term maintenance, to sustain improvement, and to prevent recurrence of symptoms." Most insurance companies refuse to cover the cost, typically $75 to $125 per treatment. Sadly, some chelationists, in an attempt to secure coverage for their patients, fraudulently present insurance claims stating they were treating heavy-metal poisoning.

More recently, two small, randomized, controlled, double-blind clinical trials of chelation therapy were published in peer-reviewed German medical journals. The first reported the results of treatment of patients suffering from arteriosclerotic obstruction of the blood supply to the lower extremities; equal improvement was noted in both the treated and control groups. The conclusion was that the improvement in walking measurements in both groups was directly attributable to the psychological effects of encouragement to increase activity. In the second trial, chelation was tested in people with coronary heart disease. Sixteen patients with angiographic (x-ray) evidence of coronary heart disease were randomized and divided into treated and untreated groups. Patients were infused with either an EDTA solution or dilute salt water (a placebo) at three-day intervals for twenty infusions. On completion, patients in both groups said they felt better, and performed weightlifting tests equally well. However, comparison of both groups before and after treatment using multiple tests found no improvement in blood flow through their coronary arteries.

Finally, the National Heart, Lung, and Blood Institute (NHLBI) sponsored a large study, which began in 2003. More than 2,300 volunteers with evidence of prior heart disease were randomized into two groups, one receiving chelation and the other receiving a placebo. The results are not expected until June 2012. The study will record many signs of arteriosclerosis, including mortality, heart attacks, strokes, and other manifestations. As there is little reason to believe chelation will prove effective, I hope that the expected results of this trial will finally resolve this controversy.

Notwithstanding the ongoing trial, virtually all mainstream medical associations agree with the American Heart Association (AHA), which stated the following: "The American Heart Association's Clinical Science Committee has reviewed the available literature on the use of chelation (EDTA) in the treatment of arteriosclerotic heart or blood vessel disease and finds no scientific evidence to demonstrate any benefit of this form of therapy. Furthermore, employment of this form of unproven treatment may deprive patients of the well-established benefits attendant to the many other valuable methods of treating these diseases." The AHA also warns of the potential dangers of chelation therapy, indicating kidney failure, bone marrow depression, shock, *hypotension* (low blood pressure), convulsions, *cardiac arrhythmias* (disturbance of heart rhythm), allergic-type reactions, and respiratory arrest. An uncertain number of deaths in the United States have been linked to chelation therapy. EDTA is approved by the FDA only for heavy metal poisoning and none of the other alleged purposes.

Why does chelation treatment continue to be promoted and performed? First, the dynamics of alternative medicine allow such treatments to persist because of the placebo effect. Extensive promotional literature also creates an aura of legitimacy. Probably the most influential book was *A Textbook on EDTA Chelation Therapy* by Elmer M. Cranton, MD, in which multiple research studies are marshaled to support the claims of its successes. Interestingly, Linus Pauling, PhD, a Nobel Prize–winning chemist, wrote the foreword of this book, having become an advocate of this technique. Although Dr. Pauling was renowned for his early scientific work, he later wandered far afield by advocating not only chelation therapy, but also massive doses of vitamin C to cure for the common cold, as well as other diseases such as cancer and heart disease. After Pauling's initial publications about vitamin C (1968–1986), subsequent scientific research, including double blind studies, has failed to support his claims in these areas. Unfortunately this renowned scientist, who died in 1994, left a controversial and sullied image for posterity.

Sadly, chelation therapy is still recommended as a treatment for many diseases. Recent Internet promotions claim success in the "reduction of fatigue, reduction of neurological symptoms (including fibromyalgia), cardiovascular symptoms, skin conditions, respiratory, gastrointestinal, genital, urinary conditions, and heavy metal poisoning (in the absence of physical symptoms)." As long as people continue to experience symptom relief following these treatments, and money is received for their execution, we will not be free of this hoax.

HOAX #2: LAETRILE

Laetrile, or laevomandelonitrile, is a trade name used for a synthetic form of amygdalin, a cyanogen compound found in the seeds of stone fruits of the *Prunus* genus (particularly apricots). Laetrile can refer to two different substances: amygdalin, which occurs naturally in apricot and peach pits and in miniscule amounts in some foods (almonds, brewer's yeast, buckwheat, sorghum, apple seeds, etc.), and synthetic Laetrile, a chemically related substance. The "laetrile" obtained in Mexico is probably in reality amygdalin.

Laetrile was first isolated in 1830 but synthesized during the early 1950s and registered with the US Patent Office for treating "disorders of intestinal fermentation." Although originally tried as an anticancer agent in Germany in 1892, it was discarded because it was deemed ineffective and excessively toxic. Much of the following discussion was based upon a review by Wilson[79] (1988).

The original purifiers of Laetrile were Ernst T. Krebs, Sr., MD, and his son Ernst, Jr. The elder Krebs, who received a medical degree in 1903, was involved in marketing Syrup Leptinol, an old Indian remedy made from parsley, which he claimed was effective against asthma, whooping cough, tuberculosis, and pneumonia. During the early 1920s, supplies of Syrup Leptinol were seized by the Food and Drug Administration (FDA) on charges that Krebs's claims were fraudulent. He was apparently not deterred; during the 1940s he and his son patented and promoted pangamic acid, later called "vitamin B15," claiming it was effective against heart disease, cancer, and other serious ailments.

The younger Krebs attended Hahnemann Medical College in Philadelphia from 1938–1939, but was expelled after failing his sophomore year. After unsuccessful attempts to secure a degree from several other colleges, he finally received a bachelor of arts degree from the University of Illinois in 1942. In 1973, he received a "doctor of science" degree from the American Christian College of Oklahoma after giving a one hour lecture on Laetrile. This college is now defunct, but had no science department and lacked authority from Oklahoma to grant doctoral degrees.

The rationale for using Laetrile to treat cancer seems to have stemmed from the work of Scottish embryologist John Beard who, in 1902, theorized that cancer cells could thrive because of the insufficiency of a pancreatic enzyme, chymotrypsin. Expanding on this convoluted logic, Krebs Jr. published a paper in 1950 claiming that Laetrile caused cancer cells to release cyanide, which destroyed these same cells without affecting normal cells. After governmental enforcement agencies began trying to ban Laetrile as a drug, Krebs claimed this drug was actually "vitamin

---

[79] Wilson B: *The rise and fall of laetrile.* Nutrition Forum 5:33-40, 1988.

B17," and that cancer results from a deficiency of this vitamin—obviously a totally preposterous claim.

One of the first practitioners to use Laetrile was Arthur T. Harris, MD, who had been a family practitioner in Southern California, but he renamed his office the "Harris Cancer Clinic." Within a year he submitted and published a report to *Coronet* magazine, claiming that he was "working on something out here that is going to be the answer to cancer if there will ever be one," but the magazine did not report what he was doing.

Having received multiple inquiries, the Cancer Commission of the California Medical Association approached Krebs Sr., who offered case reports of patients in which "spectacular results" had been observed. The commission obtained a small supply of Laetrile for animal testing at three medical centers—all of which produced negative results. Krebs' patient records were also evaluated, and no evidence of successful treatment was found.

Undaunted by these apparent failures, in 1956 Krebs Jr. enlisted the support of Andrew R.L. McNaughton, the wealthy son of the late General A.G.L. McNaughton, renowned commander of the Canadian Armed Forces during World War II. Having founded the McNaughton Foundation, which was seeking projects "on the outer limits of scientific knowledge," McNaughton began promoting and distributing Laetrile. In 1961, he founded International Biozymes Ltd. (later renamed Bioenzymes International Ltd), building factories in seven countries to manufacture Laetrile. During the 1970s, however, McNaughton became enmeshed in a financial scandal, and was charged by Italian police with having taken part in a $17 million swindle involving purchasers of Biozymes stock who falsely thought they were investing in an Italian Laetrile factory. In 1974, McNaughton was found guilty in Canada of stock fraud, fined $10,000 and sentenced to serve one day in jail. A warrant for his arrest was issued after he refused to pay the fine, and he left Canada without serving his sentence.

Despite these problems, McNaughton continued promoting Laetrile. He and Krebs Jr. managed to convince John A. Morrone, a Jersey City surgeon, to use this drug on his own patients. At McNaughton's request, Morrone wrote a report on ten patients he had treated with Laetrile, which was published in 1962 in Experimental Medicine and Surgery, a now defunct journal.

McNaughton also arranged for a freelance writer, named Glenn Kittler to produce two magazine articles and a book on Laetrile. Kittler had previously been an associate editor of Coronet magazine. His articles were published in March 1963 in American Weekly, a Sunday supplement to the Hearst newspapers. Immediately afterward, Kittler's book, carrying a foreword by McNaughton, entitled "Laetrile: Control for Cancer," was rushed into print, but when initial sales lagged, Kittler said negative pressures from the AMA and FDA were partially responsible for the anemic sales.

Given that much publicity, interest in Laetrile expanded rapidly. After reading Kittler's book in the early 1960s, a San Diego schoolteacher, Cecile Hoffman, who had suffered from breast cancer, having been unable to obtain treatments in the United States, received Laetrile treatments from a Mexican physician, Ernesto Contreras, M.D., in Tijuana. Convinced Laetrile had saved her life, she fervently supported this drug until she died of metastatic cancer in 1969. Because of her initial experience, in 1963 she formed the International Association of Cancer Victims and Friends (IACVF). This name was later changed from "Victims" to "Victors." Their purpose was "to educate the general public about the options available to cancer patients." The association began holding annual conventions in Los Angeles that drew thousands of people. These meetings provided a forum for virtually anyone who either promised or sold a cancer remedy not recognized as effective by the scientific community.

As a result of all this interest, Contreras expanded his Mexican clinic and added translators to his staff to accommodate the influx of American patients. In 1970 he constructed a new clinic—Del Mar Medical Center and Hospital—which he called "an oasis of hope." This facility is now called Oasis Hospital.

Throughout all this activity, storm clouds were gathering over Laetrile in the United States. In 1960, Laetrile was first seized from the Hoxsey Cancer Clinic, which was then operated by osteopathic physician Harry Taylor. In 1961, Krebs, Jr. and the John Beard Memorial Foundation were indicted for interstate shipment of an unapproved drug, pangamic acid (unrelated to Laetrile). After pleading guilty, Krebs was fined $3,750 and sentenced to prison. The sentence was suspended, however, when Krebs and the Foundation agreed to three-year probation during which neither would manufacture nor distribute Laetrile unless the FDA approved its use for testing as a new drug.

Despite numerous attempts during the period when Laetrile was promoted, no serious scientific studies could demonstrate that this drug affected cancer.

In 1977, a U.S. Senate subcommittee chaired by Senator Edward Kennedy held hearings on Laetrile. At these hearings, Krebs Jr. and Dr. John Richardson, a family practitioner who had prospered after becoming a "cancer expert" dispensing liberal amounts of Laetrile, claimed the FDA, AMA, NCI, American Cancer Society, and others had conspired against Laetrile. When a committee member suggested that Laetrile be tested through accepted scientific means, the respondents stated that "orthodox medicine was not qualified" to accomplish this. Senator Kennedy rightly concluded that the Laetrile promoters were "slick salesmen who would offer a false sense of hope" to cancer patients. The

New York Times commented that the Senators regarded the Laetrile promoters "with a blend of amusement and contempt."

Despite these and other governmental interventions, the saga continued to unfold. One notable event occurred in 1980, when Steve McQueen the movie star attracted considerable attention. He was treated with Laetrile at another Mexican clinic under the supervision of William D. Kelley, a dentist who had been delicensed by the State of Texas after several brushes with state and federal law enforcement authorities. Although McQueen gave a glowing report when he began his treatment, he died shortly afterward.

Finally, in response to political pressure, the National Cancer Institute responded by polling over 400,000 health professions in the United States, soliciting information about any patients who had benefitted from Laetrile. Despite the estimated 70,000 Americans who had received this drug, only sixty-eight cases were submitted for study, and, from that information, the reviewers concluded they were unable to confirm any anti-cancer activity of Laetrile.

The National Cancer Institute also undertook clinical trials in 1980, involving 178 patients at the Mayo Clinic and three other cancer centers. The results were clear: Not one patient was cured or even stabilized by laetrile. Moreover, several patients experienced symptoms of cyanide toxicity or had blood levels of cyanide approaching the lethal range. In 1980, in an accompanying editorial in the *New England Journal of Medicine*, Arnold Relman, the editor-in-chief, concluded: "Laetrile has had its day in court. The evidence, beyond reasonable doubt, is that it doesn't benefit patients with advanced cancer, and there is no reason to believe that it would be any more effective in the earlier stages of the disease . . . The time has come to close the books."

Today few sources of Laetrile are available within the United States, but it still is available at Mexican clinics and marketed as amygdalin or "vitamin B17" through the Internet.

In conclusion then, "the books" are still open—although barely—for Laetrile. As long as there are desperate patients seeking "alternatives" to scientific treatment and as long as there are charlatans ready and able to take a "fast buck," the scams will continue. Despite the recent ascendancy of groups advocating less governmental intervention at all levels, this saga contradicts these goals, affirming the role of strong governmental "watchdog" agencies dedicated protecting an often unsuspecting and uncritical public.

ALTERNATIVE MEDICINES—ADDITIONAL MYTHS AND FACTS

"The desire to take medicine is perhaps the greatest feature which distinguishes man from animals."

Sir William Osler

Of the huge number of unproven remedies on which untold quantities of money are spent, most are obtainable without a prescription from health food stores, many pharmacies, and through the Internet. Many are herbal in origin.

As you stroll through the aisles of your local health food store or pharmacy, you will be confronted with a dizzying array of complex names and competing claims. Below I provide a brief critical overview of some of the leading contenders for your attention. Hopefully this will help create order from chaos. For those who want a more comprehensive source, I would recommend R. Barker Bausell's book,[80] in which he provides a comprehensive study of a wide variety of alternative treatments. He finds no

---

[80] Bausell RB, *Snake Oil Science*. Oxford University Press. New York, N.Y., 2007.

convincing evidence that any was of real benefit. Singh and Ernst[81] reach similar conclusions in their comprehensive study, which encompassed an even broader range of alternative practices and substances.

Thus the scientific information repeatedly, and with mounting validity, points in one direction—virtually none of these treatments produces any benefit beyond the placebo effect.

Ginseng, American and Asian: Although the American and Asian types differ somewhat in structure, both are herbs, made from a root. It is promoted to counter stress, serve as a stimulant, improve the immune system, and combat ED (erectile dysfunction), among other claims. Because of differing origins and chemical structures, possible physical effects are unpredictable. American ginseng contains chemicals called *ginsenosides*, which affect the body's insulin levels. They may lower blood sugar and so possibly improve diabetic management, although blood sugar may fall to dangerously low levels if it is added to a regimen of conventional drugs.

Ginseng may include other chemicals, called polysaccharides, which may affect the immune system. Some evidence suggests that taking a specific American ginseng extract called CVT-E002 may slightly help to prevent cold or flu symptoms in adults between the ages of eighteen and sixty-five. A number of potential side effects and interactions with standard medications have been recorded, resulting in warnings to avoid ginseng during pregnancy or while taking anticoagulants (Coumadin [warfarin]), and special precautions if used with drugs to control diabetes and depression. Because of these and other risks, and since the claims of benefit are doubtful, I discourage the use of this substance.

---

[81] Singh S. and Ernst E. *Trick or Treatment: The undeniable facts about alternative medicine*. W.W. Norton Co. New York and London, 2008.

Saw Palmetto: This is the extract of the fruit of a palm tree. It appears to inhibit an enzyme that converts the hormone testosterone to an altered form called dihydrotesterone. It is best known for its use in decreasing symptoms caused by an enlarged prostate, which is called benign prostatic hypertrophy, or BPH. According to some studies, it is modestly effective for this, but improvement may not be noted for up to two months after it is started. There are standard drugs available for prostatic disorders that are likely more effective.

Other claims for its use are unproven or false. These include treating or preventing prostate infections or cancer, reducing baldness, treating upper respiratory infections such as colds, coughs, or sore throat, migraine headache, and others. In general, this product is fairly safe, but should be avoided during pregnancy or breast feeding and taken with caution when combined with female hormones, birth control pills, or any anticoagulants. Saw palmetto would best be avoided unless used for prostatic symptoms as noted.

Flaxseed Oil: Flaxseed comes from the *Linum usitatissimum* plant, and the seed's oil is used to make this product. This product has been touted to provide benefits for rheumatoid and degenerative arthritis, anxiety, BPH (benign prostatic hyperplasia), attention deficit-hyperactivity disorder (ADHD), arteriosclerosis, high blood cholesterol, and others. To date, there isn't enough scientific evidence to determine whether or not it is effective for anything. We do know, however, that it doesn't work for rheumatoid arthritis or for lowering elevated blood fats such as cholesterol and triglycerides. Although fairly safe, flaxseed oil should not be taken during pregnancy or when breast feeding. It can cause excessive bleeding when taken less than two weeks before a scheduled surgery, or when taken with other anticoagulants. I do not recommend its use.

St. John's Wort: St. John's Wort is an herb; its flowers and leaves are used to make medicine. Its name is derived from the fact that it blooms and is harvested on about June 24th, St. John's day, and "wort," an old English word for plant. The use of St. John's wort dates back to the ancient Greeks; Hippocrates recorded the medical use of its flowers.

This agent is most commonly promoted for mental depression and conditions that sometimes accompany it, such as anxiety, tiredness, loss of appetite, and trouble sleeping. Although there has been suggestive scientific evidence that it may be effective for mild to moderate depression, a more recent controlled trial[82] failed to substantiate this claim.

St. John's wort has also been tried for exhaustion, smoking cessation, fibromyalgia, chronic fatigue syndrome (CFS), migraine and other types of headaches, muscle pain, nerve pain, irritable bowel syndrome, various types of cancer, HIV/AIDS, and hepatitis C. None of these latter claims have been substantiated. Although probably safe for most people, it can cause such side effects as trouble sleeping, vivid dreams, restlessness, anxiety, irritability, stomach upset, fatigue, dry mouth, dizziness, headache, skin rash, diarrhea, and tingling. Moreover, because of unfavorable interactions with numerous drugs, I discourage its use.

Evening Primrose Oil: This oil is derived from the seed of the evening primrose plant. It is supposedly useful in treating such ailments as skin disorders, arthritis, osteoporosis (soft bones), cancer, high cholesterol, heart disease, Alzheimer's disease, schizophrenia, premenstrual syndrome (PMS), breast pain, endometriosis, symptoms of menopause including hot flashes, and others. There is no scientific evidence to justify any of these claims. In foods, evening primrose oil provides a dietary source of

---

[82] Shelton R.C., et al. *Effectiveness of St. John's Wort in major depression: A randomized controlled trial.* J.A.M.A. 2001:285; 1978-1986.

essential fatty acids. In manufacturing, evening primrose oil is used in soaps and cosmetics.

Although this agent is fairly safe for most people, there are some concerns. It should not be used during pregnancy. It should also be avoided by persons having a bleeding disorder or those taking anticoagulant medications, since it might increase the chance of bruising and bleeding. It might also increase the chance of bleeding during or after surgery, and should be discontinued at least two weeks before a scheduled operation.

There is no justification for using evening primrose oil for any medical purpose.

Melatonin: This is a natural substance normally produced in humans by the pineal gland, which is located in the center of the brain. Although not the sole regulator, it is involved in the sleep-wake cycle. Its production is inhibited by light and stimulated by darkness, which seems related to its ability to promote sleep. Medical melatonin is usually made synthetically. It is most commonly available as pills, but is also available in forms that are absorbed when placed in the cheek or under the tongue. Taken thirty to ninety minutes before bedtime, melatonin acts as a mild hypnotic, causing melatonin blood levels to rise earlier than that of the brain's own production. It appears to have some use against other sleep disorders such as jet lag, shift work, and helping blind people establish a day-and-night cycle.

Although touted for other uses against a variety of disorders ranging from cancer to headaches, these claims are unsubstantiated. It is generally safe to use, although it may aggravate depression, high blood pressure, diabetes, seizure disorders such as epilepsy, and should not be taken during pregnancy or with anticoagulants or sedatives. Its place in medicine has yet to be established, although it may be taken for minor insomnia rather than standard hypnotic (sleep-inducing) medications.

Ginkgo, also Ginkgo Biloba: This substance is extracted from the leaves of the Chinese maidenhair tree. It has been used in herbal medicines for thousands of years. The supplement, made from the leaf, is available in pills and teas. It is commonly used to help prevent Alzheimer's disease and other forms of dementia, and also to enhance memory and increase mental focus. Unfortunately, these claims are unsubstantiated, and the results of a major trial published in the *Journal of the American Medical Association* in 2008 refute its efficacy. The study, the largest ginkgo-dementia trial ever, followed more than 3,000 people age seventy-five or older for roughly six years. The supplement did not decrease the incidence of Alzheimer's disease or other dementias in people with normal cognition or those with mild cognitive impairment. Although this substance is quite safe, there is some concern about an increased risk of bruising and bleeding, as well as potential drug interactions. I advise avoiding this product.

Garlic (*Allium sativum*): This is one of the most commonly recommended herbal remedies. Although it was thought to be effective against infections, rheumatism, heart disease, diabetes, cancer, and other disorders, most studies suggest it is modestly effective only for blood pressure and cholesterol control. Some credible studies have shown that it reduces blood pressure by as much as 7–8%, and blood cholesterol levels by approximately 4–6%.

Unfortunately, there is wide variation among garlic products sold for medicinal purposes. The amount of allicin, the active ingredient and source of garlic's distinctive odor, depends on the method of preparation and the fact that it is unstable. Some manufacturers age garlic to make it odorless; unfortunately, this also reduces allicin content, and so may compromise any effectiveness.

Because of the many pitfalls in evaluation of product type, efficacy, and dosage requirements, I recommend against seeking garlic products in medicinal form and advise that you opt for the real thing. Culinary garlic is tasty, safe to use, and fits well into a Mediterranean diet, which promotes better health. It can be used to supplement the standard medications prescribed to treat elevated blood pressure and cholesterol levels. It is safe to use, provided it is ingested below levels that produce odors compromising social acceptance.

Soy: This common source of dietary phytoestrogens has weak *estrogenic* (female hormone) activity, and is commonly used to treat menopausal symptoms and to lower cholesterol. Recent systematic reviews examining the effects of increased dietary soy and soy extracts have found neither to be very effective for menopausal symptoms. Another recent review found soy effective for modestly lowering total and low-density lipoprotein (LDL), often informally called the *bad cholesterol* particles that promote cardiovascular disease, by about 4–5%, which may justify its use as a supplement to more effective means of lowering cholesterol.

Echinacea: This product supposedly treats the common cold. Although there are a limited number of controlled trials, there is no convincing evidence for efficacy. The herb is probably safe; prior studies show rates of side effects to be similar in echinacea and placebo groups. One may try it, but the cold will probably resolve within one to two weeks anyway.

ADDITIONAL NON-HERBAL ALTERNATIVES

Coenzyme Q10: This is a vitamin-like substance found naturally in the body, especially in the heart, liver, kidney, and pancreas. It resides within cells, and seems to aid in aerobic energy generation. It is present in normal diets containing meat and seafood, but is also manufactured within the body. Consequently, deficiency of this substance is rare; but nevertheless, it has been synthesized and sold for oral use as a medicine.

Multiple claims have been made for its use, including improving heart health, migraine headaches, high blood pressure, increasing energy, extending lifespan, improving the health of the gums, and many others. Some research suggests that taking coenzyme Q10 supplements might slow decline in early Parkinson's disease, but it does not seem beneficial in more advanced stages. But evidence for its benefit for other uses is conflicting or absent. Some studies suggest that, when taken along with standard medications, it may play a supporting role in improving heart function in individuals suffering from heart failure or in the months after a heart attack. Beyond this, it provides no help in controlling high blood pressure, and little evidence supports any role in preventing migraine headaches.

Overall, there is an almost total lack of evidence to support the use of coenzyme Q10. This agent seems to be safe for most adults when taken orally, but it can cause some mild side effects including stomach upset, loss of appetite, nausea, vomiting, and diarrhea. It can also cause allergic skin rashes in some people. Additionally, it may lower blood pressure more than desired, so this should be monitored. Since this agent is fairly safe, there seem to be no contraindications to its use. It could prove useful as an adjunct to standard treatment of some heart diseases, but I would discourage its use as a general tonic.

Glucosamine and Chondroitin: Glucosamine is a natural substance found in healthy human cartilage, of which it is an essential building block, as well as of ligaments, bone, and blood vessels. Considered a dietary supplement, it is available in pharmacies or health food stores and sometimes combined with another supplement, chondroitin (see below). This agent is proposed as a treatment for osteoarthritis (degenerative arthritis). Although earlier reports suggested it might be effective, more recent, carefully controlled studies have refuted this claim. Thus there is no justification for the use of this substance.

Chondroitin also occurs naturally in the body and is a component of healthy joint tissue. Supplied as pills, it is also designated as a dietary supplement. It is often combined with glucosamine, as noted above. There is no credible evidence that this substance, either alone or combined with glucosamine, has any beneficial effect.

Despite the absence of benefit of both glucosamine and chondroitin taken orally, they are often marketed together in the form of skin creams to be applied over painful joints. Needless to say, these products also fail the test of objective science, and may be about as useful as snake oil.

Magnetic Therapy and Copper Bracelets: Dating back centuries to the Greeks, Celts, Incas, and Arabs, magnetism was believed to have curative effects. No claims have ever been substantiated.

Although devoid of magnetic properties, copper, worn as bracelets or other adornments, has been advocated to treat all types of arthritis, as well as other illnesses. Such bracelets are still worn by people worldwide. Although long discredited by mainstream medicine, the myth surrounding copper bracelets was finally tested in a recent controlled study.[83] Forty-five people aged fifty or older who were diagnosed with osteoarthritis (degenerative arthritis), the most common joint problem, wore each of the following devices for four weeks during the sixteen-week study; a commercially available magnetic wrist strap; an identical strap with a weaker magnet; a de-magnetized strap; and a copper bracelet. At the start of the study and after each phase, the participants completed questionnaires indicating their pain levels, stiffness, and how easily they could do everyday tasks. No difference was found among the four devices for any of these factors.

The researchers concluded that magnetic wrist straps and copper bracelets don't help osteoarthritis symptoms, and any

---

[83] Richmond SJ. *Magnet therapy for the relief of pain and inflammation in rheumatoid arthritis (CAMBRA): A randomized placebo-controlled crossover trial.* Trials. 2008; 9: 53. Published online 2008 September 12.

improvements people perceive while using these devices are probably due to the placebo effect. My advice? Save your money.

AVOID THESE SUPPLEMENTS

The following list was formulated by Consumers Union in collaboration with the Natural Medicines Comprehensive Database. All these substances have been linked to serious side effects by clinical research or case reports.

The list includes aconite, bitter orange, chaparral, colloidal silver, coltsfoot, comfrey, country mallow, germanium, greater celandine, kava, lobelia, and yohimbe. Details about these can be obtained from the organizations noted above.

A FINAL WARNING ABOUT HERBS

Because herbs are plants, they are often considered natural, and therefore safe. However, herbs can cause undesirable effects, resulting from biologically active constituents, contaminants, and herb-drug interactions.[84] Contaminants in herbal products may be particularly problematic in medicines imported from Asia. A study investigating two-hundred-sixty Asian patent medicines found that 25% contained high levels of heavy metals, and another 7% included undeclared drugs, added purposefully and illegally to produce a desired effect.

Case reports have described serious liver and kidney damage from herb ingestion, the latter being particularly well documented. The National Kidney Foundation has identified thirty-nine herbs that may be harmful to the kidney, especially in the setting of chronic renal disease, including, among others, bucha leaves, juniper berries, St. John's wort, echinacea, ginkgo, ginger, and blue cohosh.

---

[84] Bent S. *Herbal Medicine in the United States: Review of Efficacy, Safety, and Regulation.* J. Gen Intern Med. 2008; 23: 854–859.

The safety of using most herbs with conventional drugs is largely unknown. St. John's Wort is notoriously interactive; it interferes with drugs, including chemotherapeutic agents and oral contraceptives, metabolized by a liver enzyme system.

Because many herbs contain pharmacologically active compounds, some may cause undesirable results from excessive biological effects. For example, ephedra, which contains ephedrine, an adrenaline-like substance, was widely used in traditional Chinese medicine for thousands of years. It became popular in this country in the 1990s as a component of weight-loss and energy-enhancing products. Ephedra is both a stimulant and a thermogenic (increases body heat); its biological effects are due to its ephedrine and pseudoephedrine content. These compounds stimulate the brain, increase heart rate, constrict blood vessels (increasing blood pressure), and expand bronchial tubes (making breathing easier). Their thermogenic properties cause an increase in metabolism, evidenced by an increase in body heat. Because of serious side effects, however, the FDA banned this substance on April 12, 2004. Unfortunately, it has been replaced by another herb, *Citrus aurantium* (bitter orange), which contains synephrine, which shares many of the same pharmacological properties and side effects with ephedrine.

Unfortunately, the true frequency of side effects for most herbs is unknown; they have not been tested in large clinical trials, and surveillance systems are far less rigorous than those in place for pharmaceutical products. The Office of the Inspector General conducted a review of herbal products and concluded that monitoring systems designed to detect adverse reactions are not only inadequate but probably detect less than 1% of events.[85]

The potential for toxicity from certain herbs is compounded by the frequent use of misleading marketing information. Illegal

---

[85] *Adverse event reporting for dietary supplements: An inadequate safety valve.* US:: Office of the Inspector General, HHS.; 2001.

and erroneous marketing claims for herbal products are common. In one study of Internet marketing, more than half of herbal products evaluated included false assertions that they could treat, prevent, diagnose, or cure specific diseases.[86] For example, a systematic review of *Citrus aurantium* for weight loss found only one methodologically flawed study examining its effects, which incorrectly reported a statistically significant benefit for weight loss when, in fact, the herb was no more effective than a placebo. This misleading article has been cited as published scientific evidence of the efficacy of *Citrus aurantium* for weight loss, with no mention of possible side effects.

In Europe, the situation is not much different; however, the European Union recently enacted a law that requires herbal products to be licensed or prescribed by a licensed herbal practitioner (there is no such category in the U.S.) In order for a product to be licensed, evidence for safety must be presented. This promises to improve safety, but says nothing about whether an herb is effective against any disorder it purportedly treats, affording little protection to the consumer.

THE POLITICIZATION OF ALTERNATIVE MEDICINE

The clash between myth and reality is best exemplified by the entrance of our government into the realm of alternative medicine. The Office of Alternative Medicine was founded in 1991; in 1998 it was re-established as NCCAM (National Center for Complementary and Alternative Medicine) under the auspices of the National Institutes of Health (NIH). Its mission statement states the following: "The mission of NCCAM is to define, through rigorous scientific investigation, the usefulness and safety of complementary and alternative medicine interventions and their roles in improving health and health care." This grandiose

---

[86] Morris CA, Avorn J. *Internet marketing of herbal products.* JAMA. 2003; 290:1505–9.

statement, however, does not represent what has actually transpired.

Senator Tom Harkin, a Democrat from Iowa, was instrumental in establishing NCCAM. His apparent motivation apparently resulted from a personal experience; he claimed that swallowing vast numbers of bee pollen capsules cured his allergies. This evinces misguided logic in more than one way. Using one example as a proxy for the entire world (faulty inductive reasoning) is perhaps the major flaw; the post-hoc fallacy may also have contributed, as well as the time (dis)honored belief that like can cure like (representative bias).

So, what are the lofty goals laid out by this mission statement, and what has become of them? First, we list these goals separately:

1. **Advancing scientific research**
We fund research projects at scientific institutions across the United States and around the world.

2. **Training CAM researchers**
We support training for new researchers as well as encourage experienced researchers to study CAM.

3. **Sharing news and information**
We provide timely and accurate information about CAM research in many ways, such as through our Web site, Twitter, Facebook, and other social media tools, our information clearinghouse, fact sheets, Lecture Series, and continuing medical education programs.

4. **Supporting integration of proven CAM therapies**
Our research helps the public and health professionals understand which CAM therapies have been proven to be safe and effective.

The various "therapies" to which they refer include a vast laundry list of goofy, semi-goofy, and quasi-rational practices: Homeopathy, naturopathy, traditional Chinese medicine, Ayurveda, meditation, prayer, mental healing, art therapy, music therapy, dance therapy, dietary supplements, herbal supplements, and other scientifically unproven therapies such as shark cartilage, spinal manipulation and massage, qi gong, Reiki, therapeutic touch, and electromagnetic therapy. I could probably go further, but will not try the reader's patience.

So what are the fruits of this ill-conceived department? During the 1990s, it drew increasing criticism for disdaining the scientific study of alternative approaches in favor of uncritical boosterism. Paul Berg, a Nobel Prize–winning chemist, wrote the following to the US Senate: "Quackery will always prey on the gullible and uninformed, but we should not provide it with cover from the NIH." Allen Bromley, then-president of the American Physical Society, wrote to Congress, stating that NCCAM had "emerged as an indiscriminate advocate of unconventional medicine. It has bestowed the considerable prestige of the NIH on a variety of highly dubious practices, some of which clearly violate basic laws of physics and more clearly resemble witchcraft." A *New York Times* editorial described it as "Tom Harkin's folly." Similarly, a policy forum in the journal *Science* stated, "We believe that NCCAM funds proposals of dubious merit; its research agenda is shaped more by politics than by science; and it is structured by its charter in a manner that precludes an independent review of its performance...In view of the popularity of alternative therapies, it is appropriate to evaluate the efficacy and safety of selected treatments."

Although virtually no research data have established the efficacy of any alternative medicines or procedures, NCCAM has funded clinical trials of St. John's wort, echinacea, and saw palmetto—none of which were more effective than placebo. Manufacturers, however, predictably stated the studies were flawed. Moreover, the vast majority of these firms have indicated they would continue supplying these products despite the fact that a government agency said they are ineffective.

To their credit, NCCAM is funding a study of chelation therapy for coronary artery disease, as mentioned earlier, and, hopefully, their results will finally lead to the demise of this issue.

Despite these limited benefits, over the past twenty years NCCAM has awarded funds totaling nearly $2 billion in testing such popular concepts as botanicals, distance healing, magnets, and acupuncture in an effort to benefit medical conditions such as migraine, cancer, diabetes, HIV/AIDS, and multiple sclerosis.[87] All this activity has yielded very few published reports possessing any scientific merit, and nothing that would lead to new areas of scientific medical research or treatment. This translates into a monumental waste of taxpayer money.

What is the answer? To continue allowing alternative products and procedures to be marketed under vaguely worded claims of health benefits is unsatisfactory. To continue funding NCCAM with public funds to perform research—however well designed—is also a flawed strategy, because there is no mechanism to remove such products from the market after their uselessness has been documented. The best solution, in my opinion, is to place the onus on the product manufacturers to prove both the efficacy and safety of their products through well designed, controlled studies. The results should then follow the same path for approval to the FDA, which would allow NCCAM to be eliminated. This would save taxpayer dollars and eliminate the financial drain on individuals duped into using these products. Unfortunately, given conflicting political and economic interests, this is unlikely to happen.

---

[87] Mielczareck EV and Engler B. *Measuring Mythology: Startling Concepts in NCCAM Grants.* Skeptical Inquirer, Volume 26; 2012:p.38-42.

In the absence of meaningful governmental intervention, the potential buyer of any of these products should be very cautious. Although most articles advise that one should seek the advice of a physician before obtaining any of these preparations, one must understand that most physicians also have little access to meaningful objective information, including potential dangers, upon which to base any sound advice. Unfortunately, instead of providing any tangible health benefits beyond those attained through the placebo effect, alternative medicines and procedures serve mainly to provide the hucksters and quacks a safe haven from which to operate. For an objective analysis see these two excellent websites:

Science-Based Medicine (www.sciencebasedmedicine.org)

Quackwatch (www.quackwatch.org)

ᑫᓚ *Chapter Fourteen* ᓀᓚ

VITAMINS AND OTHER NUTRIENTS—MYTHS AND FACTS

"A nickel's worth of goulash beats a five dollar can of vitamins."

Martin H. Fischer

Americans want to believe in vitamin and mineral pills. According to the *Nutrition Business Journal*, an estimated $10 billion was spent on them in 2008. Vitamins have been touted to prevent or treat a variety of disorders; however, recent studies assessing their possible benefits have yielded a flurry of disappointing results. Supplements have failed to prevent Alzheimer's disease, cancer, heart attacks, strokes, diabetes, and premature death. Other failures include heart palpitations, moodiness and other symptoms of menopause, ADHD, obsessive-compulsive disorder (OCD), and seasonal affective disorder (SAD).

Although malnutrition is uncommon, some reports indicate that up to ten percent of the U.S. population has some evidence of nutritional deficiencies—mostly for vitamins B6, D, and iron[88] Non-Hispanic black people and Mexican-Americans are more likely to be vitamin D deficient compared with others. Children and women are more likely iron deficient, and the latter group deficient in vitamin B6.

Women twenty to thirty-nine years of childbearing age have the lowest iodine levels compared with all other age groups, an important finding since iodine is important in brain development of the fetus during pregnancy. Men are at increased risk for vitamin C deficiency, and seniors for vitamin B6 or B12

---

[88] Second National Report on Biochemical Indicators of Diet and Nutrition in the U.S. Population: Center for Disease Control and Prevention, 2012.

deficiency. These findings noted above come from the Center of Disease Control's analysis from participants in the National Health and Nutrition Examination Survey data reports from 1999 through 2006. Although this does not necessarily indicate existential health problems, it points out the need for further research. Nevertheless, simple preventative measures would include increasing food sources of nutrients of potential shortage: These include meats, whole grains, vegetables, and nuts (sources of vitamin B6), fish, meat, poultry, eggs, milk, and milk products, and fortified breakfast cereals (sources of vitamin B12), orange juice, grapefruit juice, peaches, sweet red peppers, and papayas (sources of vitamin C), fish, fortified milk products and other fortified foods such as breakfast cereals and orange juice (sources of vitamin D), meat, fish, poultry, lentils and beans (sources of iron), and dairy products and grains (sources of iodine).

Multivitamins: No product can compete with a healthy, well rounded diet. Meals including fruits, vegetables, whole grains, and legumes contain fiber plus thousands of health-protective substances. Thus there is no justification for supplemental extra vitamins, with the possible exception of vitamin D, vitamin B12, and folic acid. According to Linda Van Horn, PhD, professor of preventive medicine at Northwestern University, "We have yet to see well-conducted research that categorically supports the use of vitamin and mineral supplements. Most studies show no benefit, or actual harm." Although, as noted, nutritional deficiencies can occur in unusual circumstances, national health organizations clearly indicate there is no substitute for a healthy diet. Anyone who says "I know I don't eat well, but if I pop my vitamins, I'm covered" is engaging in self-deception.

Further supporting these admonitions are the more recent results of the "Iowa Women's Health Study,"[89] which followed

---

[89] Mursu J, Robien K, Harnack LJ, et al. *Dietary supplements and mortality rate in older women.* Arch. Intern Med. 2011; 171:1625-1633.

almost 39,000 older women observed for over ten years. Surprisingly, multivitamin supplementation yielded a mortality rate modestly higher in those taking multivitamins. The findings also suggest that vitamin D (and possibly calcium) supplementation was associated with a slightly reduced mortality. As noted already, data from epidemiologic studies of this type are subject to flaws such as confounding factors and the absence of men. But the underlying and categorical message is clear. Since they provide no clear benefit, one should avoid multivitamin supplements but consider instead the possible exceptions noted below.

Vitamin D and Calcium: Vitamin D is important in bone and muscle health, nervous and immune system function, cell growth and reproduction, and moderating inflammation. It may prevent or ameliorate certain types of heart disease, arteriosclerosis, hypertension (high blood pressure), diabetes, and possibly multiple sclerosis. Some research suggests it may prevent colon cancer, and—although controversial—breast, pancreatic, and prostate cancers. It's also associated with a reduced rate of depression in older people, and greater immunity against respiratory and wound infection. It may even increase longevity under certain circumstances. A study of more than three thousand heart patients[90] disclosed that those with the highest blood levels of vitamin D were the least likely to die of any cause during nearly eight years of follow-up. Another study involving more than thirteen thousand men and women found that people with the lowest blood levels of vitamin D were 26 % more likely to die than those with the highest levels during six to twelve years of observation.

---

[90] Melamed ML, et. al. *25-hydroxyl Vitamin D Levels and the Risk of Mortality in the General Population.* Arch Intern Med. Author manuscript; available in PMC 2009 August 11.

Normally we obtain vitamin D through sun exposure and dietary intake. It is manufactured by the body, but the process requires exposure to ultraviolet light. However, given the widespread use of sunscreen to prevent skin cancer, up to 36 % of Americans are low on this vitamin. Instead of risking sun exposure, I suggest taking supplemental vitamin D. Your doctor can perform a blood test to determine whether you are deficient of this vitamin. Food sources for this vitamin are limited, although some products such as milk are fortified. Natural sources include fatty fish such as catfish, salmon, mackerel, sardines and tuna; eggs; beef liver; and cod liver oil.

The latest US recommendations for the minimum daily requirement of vitamin D, or cholecalciferol—vitamin D3, the preferred form—are 600 IU (international units) for those under 70, and 800 IU for those older, based on amounts that have slowed rates of bone loss. Persons infrequently exposed to the sun, especially the elderly, and postmenopausal women may need 800–1000 IU daily. From a review of available information, I conclude that people who get at least 700 IU of vitamin D daily and take calcium supplements have denser bones, have better muscle strength, and are likely to suffer fewer falls and fractures than those who don't. The only caution is to avoid exceeding the government's safe daily upper limit of 2,000 IU. Exceeding this amount places one at risk for various side effects, including vomiting, polyuria (excessive urination), weight loss, poor appetite, constipation, weakness, heart rhythm abnormalities, and kidney stones.

For protecting bones, vitamin D usually is combined with 600 mg of calcium, although the latter is not useful for this purpose if taken alone. If osteoporosis is already present, one should seek the advice of a physician; additional medication may be needed, such as Fosamax (alendronate).[91] In addition to enhancing bone health, calcium itself appears to be capable of reducing the risk for colon cancer if diets are supplemented with at least 700 mg daily.[92] Although some studies previously suggested that calcium alone might increase the rate of cardiovascular disease, more definitive information[93] failed to confirm this suspicion.

Vitamin E: This vitamin occurs in many foods, including vegetable oils, cereals, meat and poultry, eggs, fruits, vegetables, and wheat germ oil. It is also available as a supplement. It can be used for treating a deficiency, which is rare, but can occur in people with certain genetic disorders and very low-weight premature infants. Vitamin E has antioxidant properties (see below), which led to early enthusiasm that it might help prevent arteriosclerosis, heart attacks, and other related conditions. It became the subject of intense research, which demonstrated that it is ineffective for this use. Moreover, if taken in doses exceeding 400 IU daily, it may produce such serious side effects as increased susceptibility to stroke and higher rates of prostatic cancer.

Additional touted uses for vitamin E, including prevention and treatment of cataracts, asthma, respiratory infections, skin disorders, aging skin, sunburns, cystic fibrosis, infertility, impotence, CFS, peptic ulcers, some inherited diseases, and allergies, have shown no benefit.

Because it slows blood coagulation, vitamin E should not be used for at least two weeks before a scheduled surgical procedure. In conclusion, there is no justification for the use of supplemental vitamin E.

---

[91] Ensrud K. and Schousboe JT. *Vertebral Fractures.* New England J. Med. 2011; 364:1634-1642.

[92] Chan AT, and Giovannucci EL. *Primary Prevention of Colorectal Cancer* Gastroenterology. 2010; 138: 2029–2043.

[93] Hsia J, et al. *Calcium/vitamin D supplementation and cardiovascular events.* Circulation 2007;115:846.

Vitamin C: Vitamin C is effective in preventing and treating scurvy, the disease resulting from its deficiency. Although now rare, scurvy was once common among sailors, pirates, and others who spent long periods at sea without access to fresh fruits and vegetables. These foods, especially citrus fruits, are great sources for this vitamin and better than taking supplements. Dietary levels of about 300-400 mg/day maintain adequate body stores. One 8 ounce glass of orange juice contains about 100 mg. Fresh-squeezed juice and fresh-frozen concentrate are better than ready-to-drink forms. Reconstituted, fresh-frozen concentrate is best consumed within one week after reconstitution; ready-to-drink orange juice should be bought three to four weeks before the expiration date, and should be consumed within one week of opening. Vitamin C can also improve the body's ability to absorb iron.

Any benefits from vitamin C beyond preventing its deficiency are, at best, questionable. In the past, it was used most often for preventing and treating the common cold. Early evidence suggested that while high doses might shorten a cold's duration by about one to one-and-a-half days, it does not prevent colds. More recently, however, a pooled analysis of thirty trials involving 11,350 subjects showed that preventative use of 200 mg/day or more of vitamin C did not significantly reduce the risk of developing a cold, or of the severity of symptoms.[94]

Additional claims for vitamin C are legendary and are questionable, if not false. These include treating and/ or preventing gum disease, acne, bronchitis, HIV, stomach ulcers, tuberculosis, dysentery, bladder and prostate infections, depression, thinking problems, dementia, Alzheimer's disease, physical and mental stress, fatigue, ADHD, arteriosclerosis, high blood pressure, cataracts, gallbladder disease, dental cavities, constipation, Lyme

---

[94] Douglas RM et al. *Vitamin C for preventing and treating the common cold.* Chochrane Database Syst Rev 2007 ;(3):CD000980.

disease, skin infections producing boils (furunculosis), and many others. Skin preparations containing vitamin C, sometimes combined with other ingredients, seem to modestly improve wrinkles in facial skin aged by sun exposure.

This many claims for vitamin C probably constitute prima facie evidence that all are invalid. If this vitamin were effective as alleged for even a few of the conditions noted above, proof by rigorous testing would be available, and the entire population would be consuming it regularly—maybe from the public water supply.

Vitamin A and Beta-Carotene: Vitamin A and carotenoids, including beta-carotene, are needed by the retina for both low-light and color vision. Vitamin A also functions in a different role as an irreversibly oxidized form of retinol known as retinoic acid, an important hormone-like growth factor for skin and other cells. Beta-carotene is a potent source of vitamin A. Multivitamin preparations usually contain 1,000 to 10,000 IU (International Units) of beta-carotene. Adults and teenagers need 6 to 15 milligrams (mg) of beta-carotene (the equivalent of 10,000 to 25,000 IU of vitamin A activity) per day.

In individuals who are already at risk for lung cancer, evidence indicates that vitamin A may enhance this danger. A double-blind, randomized, placebo-controlled trial in 18,314 smokers, former smokers, and workers exposed to asbestos found that 30 mg of beta-carotene plus 25,000 IU of vitamin A taken daily for an average of four years produced a significantly increased incidence of lung cancer.[95] Similarly, a placebo-controlled trial in Finnish smokers found that 20 mg of a beta-carotene supplement significantly increased the risk of lung

---

[95] Omenn GS et al. *Effects of a combination of beta carotene and vitamin A on lung cancer and cardiovascular disease.* N England J. Med 1996; 334:1150.

cancer.[96] Additionally, one prospective study analyzing serum vitamin A levels in 29,144 men found that concentrations were associated with an increased risk of prostate cancer.[97]

Given the lack of benefit coupled with the potential risk of cancer, supplementation with vitamin A or beta-carotene is not a good idea.

Vitamin B12: This vitamin, also called cobalamin, plays a key role in the normal functioning of the brain and nervous system and blood formation. It is also involved in the metabolism of every cell of the human body, and is the largest and most structurally complicated vitamin.

Normal diets contain plentiful vitamin B12; especially rich sources are fish, meat and poultry, eggs, milk, and milk products. Although it is generally not present in plant foods, fortified breakfast cereals are a readily available source. Some nutritional yeast products also contain vitamin B12. Fortified foods vary in formulation, but product labels show which added nutrients they contain.

The daily requirement of vitamin B12 for most normal individuals is 2.5–3 micrograms. More may be needed in pregnancy or those who have intestinal disorders that interfere with its absorption. Food sources contain more than enough of this vitamin to satisfy ordinary requirements.

Vitamin B12 deficiency is common in older individuals. Atrophy of the stomach lining, which afflicts about 10–30% of the elderly, reduces the ability to absorb this vitamin from food, but such individuals can usually absorb a purified form. It can be taken

---

[96] Virtamo J. et al. *Incidence of cancer and mortality following alpha-tocopherol and beta-carotene supplementation: a post intervention follow-up.* J.A.M.A. 2003; 290:476.
[97] Mondul AM et al. *Serum retinol and risk of prostate cancer.* Am. J. Epidemiol. 2011; 173:813.

by mouth, dissolved under the tongue, sprayed into the nose, or taken monthly by intramuscular injection. Deficiency of this vitamin can lead to *pernicious anemia,* a serious form of anemia often associated with damage to the nervous system. For this reason, the elderly should consider regular B12 supplementation. If there is doubt, a blood test can indicate deficiency. Individuals most vulnerable to this deficiency are over fifty years of age, regularly taking antacids, taking metformin (for control of blood sugar), strict vegetarians, or have inflammatory bowel disease. Those falling into any of these categories should consult with a physician about blood testing.

Without evidence of its deficiency, B12 has been used for many years as a "general tonic" to combat symptoms such as fatigue and various other subjective ailments. This benefit is obtained solely through the placebo effect, enhanced by the fact that it is commonly given by injection at regular intervals, providing "hands on" administration that also increases its costs. Thus there is no justification for using B12 in this way.

Folic Acid, also called vitamin B9 or folate, is essential for numerous bodily functions, including the manufacture and repair of DNA (deoxyribonucleic acid). It promotes rapid cell division and growth as encountered in infancy and pregnancy. Children and adults both require folic acid to produce healthy blood cells and prevent anemia.

All enriched cereal grains sold in the United States contain approximately 0.140 mg of folic acid per 100 gm (about three ounces). It is also present in beans, peas, oranges, and dark-green, leafy vegetables. A standard diet provides .05–0.5 mg of this vitamin per day, which is adequate for normal individuals. However, even a generous intake of these foods may not provide enough folic acid to prevent certain birth defects (neural tube defects) during pregnancy, which may occur before most women are aware that they are pregnant. This provides an incentive for folic acid supplementation in all women of child-bearing age. Such women may consider supplementing with 0.8 mg daily. The oral form of folic acid, taken as a supplement, is usually absorbed better than that found naturally in food.

Although generally non-toxic, when folic acid is taken alone, it may exacerbate problems associated with vitamin B12 deficiency, which can lead to malfunctioning of the nervous system. Thus anyone at risk for B12 deficiency should not begin supplementation with folic acid alone without consulting a physician.

Folic acid provides an interesting example of why apparently good ideas require objective scientific testing. Elevated blood levels of *homocysteine*, a non-protein amino acid produced by the body, are associated with excessive risk for heart and vascular disease. Logic dictates that reduction of this substance in the blood might produce a breakthrough in the reduction of cardiovascular disorders. Folic acid, along with vitamins B6 and B12, can reduce blood levels of homocysteine to normal. Unfortunately, the expected parallel reduction in disease does not occur. In randomized, double-blind, placebo-controlled trials, large doses of folic acid, vitamin B6 (pyridoxine), and vitamin B12, given for periods up to five years, reduced homocysteine levels, but had no effect on the incidence of cardiovascular disorders.[98] This again demonstrates the danger of assuming that association means causation.

Fish Oil: This product consists of the omega-3 fatty acids eicosapentaenoic acid (EPA) and docosahexaenoic acid (DHA). They are especially prevalent in oily fish such as trout, mackerel, sardines, salmon, anchovies, and herring. Including these types of

---

[98] Ebbing M. et. al. *Combined analyses and extended follow-up of two randomized controlled homocysteine-lowering B-vitamin trials.* J. Intern Med 2010; 268:367.

fish once or twice weekly in one's diet retards the process of arteriosclerosis.

These oils are available in purified form, and although slight differences in biological activity exist between EPA and DHA, both exert several positive actions against atherosclerosis and its complications.[99] They reduce blood *triglycerides* (a fatty substance linked to arteriosclerosis) while leaving other blood fats essentially unaltered. They also affect platelets, essential to blood clotting, which reduces the tendency for blood to clot and thus potentially reduces the threat of heart attack and other conditions. They lower blood pressure slightly, may combat depression, and mildly reduce certain heart rhythm irregularities. Two large studies have shown that fish oils can reduce the frequency of sudden cardiac death or major adverse cardiac events.

Krill oil supplements also supply omega-3 fatty acids, but this oil comes from small crustaceans, not fatty fish, and it contains more EPA, possibly providing an advantage for this latter substance. Krill supplements are likely safe, and obtainable in drugstores, health-food stores, and online. The price per pill is often around thirty cents, approximating that of some fish-oil capsules. Some preliminary research suggests that this substance may have anti-inflammatory properties, reducing symptoms from arthritis and even pre-menstrual distress. More definitive research, however, will be needed to confirm this hypothesis and how this substance compares with fish oil in the promotion of heart health.

Evidence from large trials suggests that EPA+DHA supplementation ranging from 0.5 to 1.8 g/d (either as fatty fish or supplements) significantly reduces subsequent cardiac and all-cause mortality. A growing body of evidence also indicates that α-linolenic acid, a vegetable oil similar to fish oil, is associated with

---

[99] Kris-Etherton PM, Harris WS, and Appel LJ. Fish Consumption, Fish Oil, Omega-3 Fatty Acids, and Cardiovascular Disease *Circulation. 2002; 106: 2747-2757.*

a lower risk of these diseases in women and in men. For α-linolenic acid, total intakes of 1.5 to 3 g/d seem to be beneficial. These data support inclusion of vegetable oils (e.g., soybean, canola, walnut, and flaxseed) and food sources (e.g., walnuts, flaxseeds) high in α-linolenic acid in a healthy diet for the general population. Many over-the-counter preparations of these purified oils are available.

Cautions concerning fish products: Although generally quite safe, doses of fish oil can be problematic, for about a third of people taking 3 grams or more a day develop abdominal pain, belching, bad breath or an unpleasant fishy taste in their mouths. Otherwise this product is safe and is free of contaminants such as mercury. Some species of fish, however, may contain significant levels of methylmercury, polychlorinated biphenyls (PCBs), dioxins, and other environmental contaminants. These substances are present at low levels in fresh waters and oceans, and they bioconcentrate in the aquatic food chain such that levels are generally highest in older, larger, predatory fish. Children and pregnant and lactating women may be at increased risk for mercury intoxication from fish consumption. Thus, this group should minimize such potentially contaminated fish. For middle-aged and older men and postmenopausal women, the benefits of fish consumption far outweigh the risks.

Fish allergies are occasionally encountered, and these products must be avoided in susceptible individuals. Symptoms of allergy to fish oil are the same as those reactions to fish. Although most fish oil supplements are free of allergy-causing fish proteins, molecules from some of the fish proteins may be present. Thus a patient with a known fish allergy should avoid the use of fish oil supplements

ANTIOXIDANTS: A NEW ENTRANT IN "THE HOAX PARADE"

During the past ten years, *antioxidant* has become the buzzword du jour, used to describe agents that combat the process of oxidation. Originally applied to preventing the oxidation of metals, such as the rusting of iron, and later extended to averting rancidity in foods, the meaning of this word has recently been extended to the study of cellular physiology in living tissue (suspiciously reminiscent of the representative bias).

Early research demonstrated that the process of oxidation within the body's cells could lead to the formation of *free radicals*, or molecules capable of producing damage as the body breaks down food or is exposed to environmental irritants, like tobacco smoke and radiation. This led to the hypothesis that interruption of this process could reduce cell damage and, hopefully, promote better health. For instance, early studies suggested that the interruption of oxidation may slow or possibly prevent cancer and arteriosclerosis, the latter because the oxidation of low-density lipoprotein (LDL, or bad) cholesterol is important in developing fatty buildups in the arteries, which can lead to heart attacks and strokes. Until recently, evidence suggested that oxidation of LDL cholesterol and its presumably harmful biological effects could be prevented by using antioxidant supplements such as vitamin E. More recent clinical trials, however, have failed to confirm this hypothesis. They have also failed to show that these supplements prevent cancer or help treating it. As noted previously, vitamin E turned out to be a dismal flop.

Chemical analyses have uncovered the existence of many antioxidants occurring in normal diets and in vitamin supplements. What are these agents, and can they improve human health?

Antioxidants are abundant in fruits and vegetables, as well as nuts and grains, and some meats, poultry, and fish. Food sources of common antioxidants are listed below.

1. Alpha- and beta-carotene are found in many orange-colored foods, such as sweet potatoes, carrots, cantaloupe, squash, apricots, pumpkin, and mangos. Some green, leafy vegetables, including spinach, broccoli, green beans, turnip greens, collards, leaf lettuce, and kale, are also rich in these carotenes.

2. Lutein is abundant in green, leafy vegetables.

3. Lycopene, a potent antioxidant, is found in tomatoes, watermelon, guava, papaya, apricots, pink grapefruit, and blood oranges, among others.

4. Selenium, a mineral that supports antioxidant processes, is contained in rice and wheat.

Antioxidant vitamins, including C, E, and the carotenes, have been subjected to intensive study for potential general health-promoting properties. Focus on the carotenes has been intense, and in a recent large study,[100] higher blood levels of alpha-carotene were associated with lower death rates related to cancer, diabetes, and certain respiratory disorders. This relationship seems to be specific to alpha-carotene, which is obtained mainly through the diet and not usually a part of artificial supplements or food additives. By contrast, supplementation of diets with beta carotene has shown no benefit for the general population, and it may even increase one's risk for cancer. In conclusion, the belief that antioxidant supplements are beneficial seems to be erroneous for, paradoxically, oxidation may actually be one of the keys to extension of our life span.[101] Overall, these findings emphasize the

---

[100] Chaoyang L, Ford ES, Zhao G. et. al. *Serum alpha-carotene concentrations and risk of death among US adults.* Arch. Internal Medicine. 2011; 171:507-513.
[101] Park S, Murphy SP, Wilkens LR, et al. *Multivitamin use and the risk of mortality and cancer incidence: the multiethnic cohort study.* Am. J. Epidemiology. 2011; 173:906-914.

importance of good diet in preference to various dietary supplements.

What has come of all this speculation about antioxidants? Regarding dietary composition, all the foods listed above have been demonstrated to promote overall health, including reduction of heart disease and certain types of cancer. Regardless of whether or not diets have antioxidant properties, there are better reasons for their success, including fiber content, cholesterol reduction, and a fairly large potassium content, which has been shown to help control proper levels of blood pressure and reducing mortality possibly through other possible means.[102] Thus there is no credible evidence to support the routine use of antioxidant supplements for these purposes.

In conclusion, don't fall for a hokey term like antioxidant, which is designed to separate you from your money. There is no substitute for a good, healthy, and well-rounded diet. The subject was summarized nicely by science writer Sharon Begley, in the January 25, 2011 issue of *Newsweek*. In her article, titled "Antioxidants Fall from Grace," she not only reviews evidence showing these agents produce no health benefits, but also quotes Jeffrey Blumberg, director of the Antioxidants Research Lab at Tufts University, who says that antioxidants "are believed to initiate, promote, or stimulate the progression of many chronic diseases, including cardiovascular disease and cancer, as well as normal aging." Backing up these contentions, the position of the ACS, the National Cancer Institute (NCI), and several international health organizations is that antioxidants—if effective at all— should come from a healthy diet, not from dietary supplements. The AHA also cautions against using antioxidant vitamin supplements "until more complete data are available."

---

[102] Yang Q, Liu T, Kuklina EV, et. al. *Sodium and potassium intake and mortality among US adults*. Arch. Int. Med. 2011; 171:1183-1190.

Not surprisingly, the *Newsweek* article triggered a firestorm of protest, including numerous irate Internet postings, some of which came from sources that stand to gain financially from selling and promoting these products. For instance, a spokesman for the Alliance for Natural Health, an organization promoting alternative medicine, responded with a long-winded and arcane theoretical discussion about the presumed shortcomings of this article, but no research data were offered to support any counter arguments—a usual smokescreen thrown up by such organizations, aimed at obfuscation rather than elucidation. Their argument concluded by stating "for likely the next decade at least, be very skeptical of health advice offered by *Newsweek* or any of the mainstream media, particularly if it's about the natural approach to healthcare." No further comment is required.

ᴄᴘ *Chapter Fifteen* ᴄ◌

NUTRITION AND WEIGHT REDUCTION: FACTS AND MYTHS

"At the end of every diet, the path curves back toward the trough."

Mason Cooley

Probably the greatest myths and confusion surround the issues of food and dietary supplements. The best source for authoritative answers to most questions on this subject can be found in *Consumer Reports (Health)* but definitely not from sensational reports found in check-out-counter tabloids. In this section, I will tackle some of the most important and common misconceptions about diets after providing some factual information about nutrition.

DIET AND WEIGHT REDUCTION: The tremendous impact of diet and weight reduction in our society is found everywhere—on the weekly the best-selling book lists, newsstands, or at cocktail parties. For the best overall advice about the general principles of proper nutrition and weight reduction, see *"The Volumetrics Eating Plan"* by Barbara Rolls, PhD. Weight Watchers and Jenny Craig also provide good advice.

The basic concepts of weight reduction are simple but, as we know, hard to implement: consume fewer calories than you burn. Taking in 500 fewer calories every day will result in losing about a pound a week. Additional tips include not skipping breakfast and restricting fat intake, especially bad fats (*trans fats* and saturated fats). Good fats include olive and other monounsaturated oils, nuts, avocados, and omega-3 oils from seafood and plant sources. However, all fats are calorie rich and, if eaten in excess, will make weight reduction more difficult.

Healthy diets consist of plenty of fruits and vegetables, and some lean meat and fish, fats derived from vegetable or fish sources, and whole grains; they minimize refined grains, potatoes, and full-fat dairy products. Soft drinks are discouraged. Even if one substitutes for these drinks with low calorie versions, evidence suggests—for reasons that are unclear—they may actually promote cardiovascular risk. Studies of large populations worldwide show that these overall eating patterns reduce the risk of heart disease, diabetes, and certain cancers and, when moderate quantities are consumed, obesity.

Regarding the prevention of heart disease and arteriosclerosis, Mozaffarian et al.[103] have recently provided comprehensive, scientifically grounded guidance. The authors emphasize the importance of natural foods, stating that "benefits do not appear reproducible with equivalent amounts of representative mineral and fiber supplements, nor are they dependent on dietary macronutrient (fat, protein, or carbohydrate) composition." They group all fruits and vegetables together, stating that "potential differences in health effects contributed by specific types of fruits, vegetables, or their juices require further investigation," and emphasize the importance of whole grains, meaning primarily bran, germ, and endosperm from natural cereal. The authors point out that regular fish consumption can reduce mortality from heart disease by approximately 36%, but caution that consumption of commercially fried fish or fish sandwiches has not shown these benefits for reasons that are unclear. Tree nuts and peanuts seem to combat cardiovascular disease through several mechanisms, but the effects of specific types require further study.

Regarding red meats, they noted that consumption of processed meats (e.g., hot dogs, lunch meat, etc.) seemed to

---

[103] Mozaffarian D., Appel LJ, and Van Horn L. *Components of a Cardioprotective Diet. New Insights. Circulation* (American Heart Association). 2011; 123:2870-2891.

possess the highest risk of heart disease and diabetes, suggesting that preservatives (sodium, nitrites, and phosphates and/or preparation methods) could adversely influence the health effects of meat consumption. Even unprocessed meats appear to carry at least modestly elevated risk for both cardiovascular disease and cancer:[104] Review of prospective studies of 37,698 man from the health professionals follow-up study (1966-2008) and 83,644 women from the nurses' health study (1980-2008) disclosed that the hazard ratio of total mortality for a 1-serving per-day increase was 1.13 for unprocessed red meat and 1.20 for processed red meat. For cardiovascular mortality, these ratios were 1.18 and 1.21, respectively, and for cancer deaths, 1.10 and 1.16. These latter authors estimated that substitutions of other foods (including fish, poultry, nuts and legumes, low-fat dairy and whole grains) for 1 serving per day of red meat would likely yield a 7% to 19% lower mortality risk. They also estimated that 9.3% of deaths in men and 7.6% in women could be prevented at the end of follow-up if all the individuals consumed fewer than 0.5 servings per day (approximately 42 gm/day) of red meat. The types of cancer were not specified, but the authors cited evidence that pointed toward colorectal cancers as the most prevalent in association with red meat.

Light or moderate alcohol consumption (up to two drinks per day for men, 1 for women) reduces cardiovascular risk, but higher consumption may increase long-term risks for cardiovascular and other diseases. Scientific evidence implicates alcohol per se in this beneficial effect. Although there is a mystique surrounding red wine, evidence fails to support that this drink possesses any properties that are superior to the alcohol it contains. Finally, these reviewers indicate that Mediterranean diets, which emphasize vegetables, fruits, breads, cereal, and foods made from wheat, nuts, and olive oil—often including fish and wine—

---

[104] Pan A, Sun Q, Bernstein AM, Schulze MB, Manson JE, Stampfer MJ, Willett WC., and Hu FB. Red meat consumption and mortality. Arch Intern Med. 2012;172:555-563.

counteract these diseases. In general, vegetarian diets exhibit similar favorable effects.

Dietary fat consumption has traditionally been linked to cardiovascular disease; however, recent evidence has raised some doubts about this issue.[105] Certainly trans fats, produced by partially hydrogenating vegetable oil, are harmful and should be reduced as much as possible. Higher consumption of saturated fats, derived from animal sources, and cholesterol has traditionally been associated with increased cardiovascular risk. This latter concept is now being challenged. Evidence now suggests that the overall diet may play a greater role in producing these potentially adverse effects. In other words, high saturated fat consumption may often be combined with other unfavorable elements, such as less-healthful refined carbohydrates which have their own detrimental effects. Thus harmful effects may be attributable to many factors beyond the ingestion of saturated fats or cholesterol. Continuing research is required to sort out these apparently conflicting factors.

Virtually all diets restrict bad, or highly refined, carbohydrates (carbs) such as white bread, cookies, chips, and sugar-sweetened soft drinks, but encourage the substitution of whole-grain, high quality carbohydrates. I do not recommend a wholesale cutback on grains, fruits, and sweeter vegetables, such as beets and carrots, which was first popularized by the Atkins diet. Recent research has demonstrated that, for up to a year, some people can indeed safely lose weight on the Atkins diet, but after this period weight loss is no better than with a conventional diet. Another downside of extreme cutbacks of carbohydrates is their effect on mental function. In one study, women who followed a carb-free diet for a week showed memory impairment when compared to those who adhered to a more balanced, reduced-

---

[105] Mozaffarian D., Appel LJ, and Van Horn L. *Components of a Cardioprotective Diet. New Insights.* Circulation (American Heart Association). 2011; 123:2870-2891.

calorie plan. This impairment was reversed quickly after resuming a normal diet. Certain negative mental effects resulting from carbohydrate restriction, however, seem to persist for longer periods. One study showed that mood disorders were more likely in those who continue on extreme low-carb diets.[106] So if you're considering such a diet, look for one that allows for some complex carbohydrates in the form of fruits, vegetables, and whole grains. That might help mitigate crankiness or brain fog.

If one's diet contains a greater proportion of low energy-density foods—foods with fewer calories per bite—calories can be spared while still eating a satisfying amount of food. Begin meals with a low-calorie soup or salad, followed by main dishes that contain liberal quantities of vegetables and fruits. Using government food consumption surveys, researcher Barbara Rolls has shown that people who eat a low energy-density diet consume hundreds fewer calories per day, which allows the former group to eat a greater volume of food, lose weight, and remain thinner.

Proper dietary habits can also prevent or aid the control of high blood pressure, and can enhance the effect of medications already being used for this purpose. Unfortunately, hypertension is far too common, affecting approximately a third of the adult population in the United States. It is a major cause of cardiovascular disease, including strokes and heart attacks. Increased salt, or sodium, intake is a major culprit in producing hypertension, and most Americans ingest far too much of it. A good general diet with reduced sodium intake—ideally less than 1,500 mg daily—is very healthy indeed. This is the DASH diet (Dietary Approaches to Stop Hypertension) but, since it contains all the elements of a good diet, it goes far beyond this goal, and may even be used for weight reduction.

---

[106] Consumer Reports on Health, October, 2011, p.8.

A detailed presentation of this diet which is well worth reading can be found in the NIH publication *Your Guide to Lowering Your Blood Pressure with DASH.* It available on the web at:

www.nhlbi.nih.gov/health/public/heart/hbp/dash/newdash.pdf

The relationship between diet and cancer prevention is of great interest. In the United States, colon cancer is the third leading cause of cancer death. In 2009, an estimated 146,970 men and women were newly diagnosed with colon and rectal cancer, with 49,920 deaths. At current rates, approximately 5%—6% of the U.S. population will develop cancer of the colon or rectum within their lifetime.[107] Evidence indicates that the Western diet is a strong contributor to this disease. Several studies have shown that not only a high intake of red and processed meats (noted above), but also highly refined grains and starches and sugars is related to an increased risk of colorectal cancer. Moreover, obesity increases the risk for these malignancies. Convincing evidence also links higher levels of body fat to an increased risk of cancers of the esophagus, pancreas, breast (postmenopausal), uterus, and kidney.[108]

The most successful way to reduce weight and keep it off is to adopt the lifestyle principles enumerated above on a continuing basis. Initial weight reduction is best achieved gradually by losing about one to two pounds per week. Crash diets, such as pre-prepared foods or temporary severe reductions of food intake may be successful in the short run but, unless overall dietary and lifestyle changes are adopted, individuals usually return to their original weight within one to two years.

---

[107] Chan AT, and Giovannucci EL. *Primary Prevention of Colorectal Cancer* Gastroenterology. 2010; 138: 2029–2043.

[108] World Cancer Research Fund/American Institute for Cancer Research. *Food, nutrition, physical activity, and the prevention of cancer: a global perspective.* Washington DC: AICR; 2007.

Regular exercise should accompany good diet, but weight control by exercise alone is virtually impossible. However, an active lifestyle will help maintain weight loss. Everyone should attempt to get sixty to ninety minutes a day of moderate to vigorous exercise such as brisk walking, jogging, aerobic sports, or some other activity you enjoy. Even lesser amounts of exercise via such activities as house and yard work help burn some calories. Apart from assisting in weight control, exercise clearly lowers the risk of cardiovascular disease and has been shown to provide at least partial protection against cancers of the colon, breast (postmenopausal), and uterus.

Before concluding this section, I must attempt to answer the currently popular question: are there any health benefits from eating organic foods? In a recent and extensive review of this subject, Dangour et al.[109] concluded that there is no evidence of any benefit from eating organically produced food. These authors concede that there is a paucity of good research on the subject, identifying only twelve relevant, well-conducted trials. So since the evidence is incomplete, the jury is still out. Given that the controversy about organic food dates back to the 1950s, it is surprising that so little good research has been done since then. However, if one considers the available studies, evidence is lacking to support claims of better nutrient quality in organically than conventionally produced foods.

The issue of pesticides, hormones, and antibiotics is tangential to the subject of organic foods. There are indeed lower levels of these synthetic agents in organic produce than in conventionally grown equivalents, but does that render it safer to consume? In the review cited above, the authors found no evidence of greater safety of organic food.

---

[109] Dangour AD, Lock K., Hayter A, et al. *Nutrition-related health effects of organic foods.* Am. J. Clin. Nutrition. 2010; 92:203.

One additional caveat about pesticides is that organic farming may employ organic, but not synthetic, pesticides, such as a rotenone-pyrethrin mixture, which has not been as well studied as synthetic pesticides. This combination often requires multiple applications and may persist in soil longer than synthetics. Thus, the use of natural pesticides is probably nothing more than an appeal to the naturalistic fantasy. Although definitive studies are lacking, there is no evidence of superior safety.

Human exposure to pesticides should always be minimized. This is easily accomplished by washing all produce thoroughly prior to consumption. Although direct comparisons of the presence of pesticide residue in organic produce vs. thoroughly washed conventional produce are lacking, residue levels are generally below safety limits, and can be lowered further by washing.

This subject, however, requires continued monitoring and further research. In conclusion, avoid the organic label, since these products lack clear benefits and are generally more expensive.

✑ *Chapter Sixteen* ✑

HOW TO AVOID FRAUDS AND RIPOFFS

"Fraud and falsehood only dread examination. Truth invites it."

Samuel Johnson

New health frauds pop up continuously, but promoters usually fall back on the same old clichés and tricks to gain your trust and get your money. NCCAM cites the following four points as red flags.

1. The vendor or practitioner claims the treatment or product works by a secret formula. Legitimate scientists share their knowledge so their peers can review the data.

2. The treatment is supposedly an amazing or miraculous breakthrough or cure. Real medical breakthroughs are few and far between, and when they happen, are not touted as amazing or miraculous by any responsible scientist or journalist.

3. The treatment is publicized only in the back pages of magazines, over the phone, by direct mail, in newspaper ads pretending to be news stories, or on thirty-minute, talk-show-format infomercials. The results of studies on bona fide treatments are generally reported first in peer-reviewed medical journals.

4. Proof for the treatment relies solely on testimonials from satisfied customers. These people may never have had the disease the product is supposed to cure, may be paid representatives, or may simply not exist. Often they're identified only by initials or first names.

As I was researching this section, I saw a large advertisement in a local newspaper which looked like a news story, except for a tiny insert at the top which read "Paid Advertisement." The article was titled "Powerful Joint Pill Flying off Drug Store Shelves." This joint pill, Trigosamine, is a combination of two old drugs, hyaluronate-13 and glucosamine sulfate-15 (see below), along with rapidflex formula-61. The latter contains "patented ingredients" that "increase the speed in which nutrients are absorbed." Interestingly, the company footnotes its claims with the following familiar statement that the product "has not been evaluated by the Food and Drug Administration. This product is not intended to diagnose, treat, cure or prevent any disease."

They go on to claim that "a team of scientists has delivered an amazing joint health supplement that's been clinically shown to improve mobility and joint comfort." Basing this claim on an alleged 8-week clinical study of fifty-four participants, they state that "On day six of the study, those participants taking Trigosamine reported statistically significant improvement in joint comfort..." Needless to say, this "study" was not evaluated in peer-reviewed medical journals. In the ad, the company's "Director of Health Science, Research Development," Dr. Wm. James (true name withheld), is a PhD (not an MD), states, "I've never seen relief like this before." There is a further statement by Dr. Raymond Heath (true name withheld), who claims, "I am thoroughly impressed with the clinical data, in fact I now take the pill myself to get the joint relief I need. It's my number one recommendation to anyone who suffers with joint discomfort." This person is an emergency room physician and medical consultant to the same company, and "remunerated for his services."

Let's examine this "miracle breakthrough." First, research results for hyaluronic acid are conflicting, but it is only of some use when injected directly into an arthritic joint by a healthcare provider. There is no evidence it is effective when taken orally. The next ingredient, glucosamine sulfate, was earlier thought somewhat effective in relieving pain from osteoarthritis but, as already discussed, subsequent studies have failed to show any benefit.[110] Finally, my efforts to determine the nature of "rapidflex formula-61," a "patented" (secret?) ingredient, were unsuccessful, suggesting the strong likelihood of a scam.

Thus the facts indicate this breakthrough treatment for joint pains or arthritis qualifies as a fraud and/or rip-off. Since I encountered this advertisement, I have seen many similar ads which make all sorts of similarly vague claims.

In conclusion, when considering over-the-counter alternative agents claiming to ameliorate or cure diseases or pains, be highly skeptical. Read the small print, which is not only revealing, but also entertaining. When there is little or no scientific evidence to support a claim, the agent in question is usually ineffective, sometimes dangerous, and regularly accompanied by the tipoff statement "...has not been evaluated by the Food and Drug Administration. This product is not intended to diagnose, treat, cure or prevent any disease." Avoid them all. At best, you are wasting your money.

We should heed the advice of Singh and Ernst,[111] who suggest labeling most of these products, including chiropractic and acupuncture therapy, with the following statement, which I have modified: "Warning: this product is a placebo. It will work only if you believe in it, and only for certain conditions which respond to placebo treatments. Even then, the placebo effect is unpredictable, and it is not likely to be as powerful as orthodox drugs or treatments. You may get fewer adverse effects from this treatment than from a standard method, but you will probably also receive less benefit." Although accurately stated, I suspect the results of

---

[110] Reichenbach S., et al. *Meta-analysis: Chondroitin for osteoarthritis of the knee or hip.* Annals of Internal Medicine, 2007; 146:580-590.
[111] Singh S. and Ernst E. *Trick or Treatment: The undeniable facts about alternative medicine.* W.W. Norton Co. New York and London, 2008.

such a warning would be no more effective than those nasty labels on cigarette packs. But who knows?

⟨ƒ⟩ *Chapter Seventeen* ⟨⟩

THE EVOLUTION OF MODERN MEDICAL CARE

"It isn't what we don't know that gives us trouble, it's what we know that ain't so."

Will Rogers

The early history of medical science is, in a sense, alternative medicine. There were very limited means available to evaluate disease and virtually no effective methods of treatment. Proposed treatments were either worthless or dangerous. Given this background, how did the public tolerate such abysmal mismanagement for so many centuries? The answer is that any treatment followed by improvement would have been attributed to that intervention, thus allowing for the post hoc ergo propter hoc fallacy. Any apparent or actual improvement in illness could have resulted from the placebo effect or from spontaneous resolution. Moreover, since many diseases fluctuate in severity, any intervention during a severe phase might be followed by a more typical milder phase, attributable to the regression-toward-the-mean fallacy. Even the confirmation bias undoubtedly played a role, for practitioners would likely have selected examples of "cures" that confirmed their preexisting ideas of acceptable treatments. The number and variety of treatments throughout the ages are legendary—prescriptions used throughout antiquity number 15,000–20,000.[112] More interesting were the physical or mechanical procedures used by caregivers, including purging, cutting, blistering, freezing, heating, sweating, leeching, and bleeding.

---

[112] Shapiro AK and Shapiro E. *The powerful placebo: from ancient priest to modern physician.* Johns Hopkins University Press, Baltimore, MD (1997).

The origin of bloodletting is difficult to trace, but was used for thousands of years to treat hysteria, heart disease, and just about every other imaginable malady. The theory behind the practice changed over time, but the practice remained the same with doctors bleeding patients, often until they were weak, pale, and sometimes unconscious. In Asia and the Mideast, patients were bled to "release demons and bad energy"; in ancient Greece, to restore the body's "balance of fluids"; in medieval and Renaissance Europe, to reduce "inflammation," then thought to be the root of all disease. Practitioners also bled patients preventatively of offset the effects of excess food, weather changes, and wounds.

By the late 1700s, bloodletting was the treatment of choice in America too, thanks partly to Founding Father, physician, writer, educator, and humanitarian Benjamin Rush, a signer of the Declaration of Independence. He believed that "tension" in blood vessels caused disease. When George Washington fell ill with an upper respiratory infection, his physicians bled him heavily, resulting in loss of more than two liters (approximately two quarts) of blood. Washington died a day later. Although historians dispute whether blood loss or complications killed him, he would obviously have been better off unbled or given chicken soup.

In the next century, physicians learned that bacteria, or germs— not an imbalance of fluids—caused most infectious diseases. Bloodletting finally disappeared by the 20th century.

Despite the primitive state of medicine before the latter part of the 19th century, glimmers of hope began to appear. Careful observers who were willing to step beyond the conventional wisdom of the time began to forge new frontiers. They were keen observers and intellects who undertook objective analysis, avoiding premature conclusions. A few notable representatives are:

Antony van Leeuwenhoek (1632–1723), the Father of Microbiology, was a Dutchman who learned to grind optic lenses, made simple microscopes, and began observing with them. Although microscopes had been in use for some 70 years, his skills enabled him to build instruments that magnified over two-hundred times with clearer and brighter images. Through careful and painstaking observation, he described such organisms as plant structures, muscle cells, red blood cells, sperm cells, protozoa (one-celled organisms) and, most notably, bacteria. He was the first to observe these latter organisms, which he called "very little animalcules." Although these were yet to be connected with diseases, his observations helped lay the foundations of modern bacteriology. What is especially revealing about Leeuwenhoek is contained in a letter he wrote in June 12, 1716.

> *"My work, which I've done for a long time, was not pursued in order to gain the praise I now enjoy, but chiefly from a craving after knowledge, which I notice resides in me more than in most other men. And therewithal, whenever I found out anything remarkable, I have thought it my duty to put down my discovery on paper, so that all ingenious people might be informed thereof."*

We can all derive inspiration from this simple—and dignified—statement.

No story better exemplifies the elegance and simplicity of the scientific approach better than that of **Edward Jenner** (1749–1823) and his conquest of smallpox.[113]

Throughout the ages, smallpox, now known to be caused by a virus, was a serious, and often deadly, disease that had spread worldwide. It appeared in Europe sometime between the 5th and 7th centuries AD, and was frequently epidemic during the Middle Ages. The fatality rate varied from 20% to 60%, and left most survivors with disfiguring scars. The medical term for smallpox

---

[113] Riedel S. Edward Jenner and the history of smallpox and vaccination Proc (Bayl Univ Med Cent). 2005:18; 21–25.

was *variola*, from the Latin *varus* meaning "mark on the skin," and *pocke*, meaning sac.

It had been known for a long time that survivors of smallpox became immune to the disease. Stemming from this observation, deliberate transmission of small amounts of infected material were taken from those with disease and transferred to those who were not immune. This was usually accomplished by rubbing material from a smallpox pustule into a scratch between the thumb and forefinger of a healthy individual, and this usually produced a milder form of smallpox, causing permanent immunity. These first inoculations, a term derived from the Latin *inoculare*, meaning "to graft." Referring to smallpox this procedure was called *variolation*. The procedure reached England in 1715, and thereafter rapidly gained popularity throughout Europe. Although still a threat, variolation produced a fatality rate ten times lower than that of naturally occurring smallpox.

Variolation reached the New World by 1721. When a ship from the West Indies carried persons sick with smallpox into Massachusetts in 1721, an epidemic broke out in Boston and other parts of the state. In response, Rev. Cotton Mather (1663–1728), and Dr. Zabdiel Boylston (1679–1766) started a variolation program. After noting that half of Boston's 12,000 inhabitants had contracted the disease, they calculated the fatality rate for the naturally contracted disease was 14%, but only 2% among variolated individuals. This may have been the first time that comparative analysis was used to evaluate a medical procedure, simulating the controlled studies that are now standard.

Jenner was born in Gloucestershire, England in 1749. When he was thirteen, he was apprenticed to a country surgeon and apothecary where he heard a dairymaid say, "I shall never have smallpox for I have had cowpox. I shall never have an ugly pockmarked face." At that time it was a common belief that dairymaids were protected from smallpox.

Having completed a surgical apprenticeship, he turned his attention to smallpox in 1796 and began the process that culminated in the worldwide eradication of this disease. Remembering the dairymaid's statement, he hypothesized that immunity to cowpox might confer immunity to smallpox, and then postulated that transmitting cowpox from one person to another might confer immunity against smallpox. In May 1796, Jenner inoculated an eight-year-old boy with matter from a dairymaid's cowpox lesion. The boy developed a mild fever and some discomfort, but recovered within ten days after the procedure. In July, Jenner inoculated the boy with matter from a fresh smallpox lesion. No disease developed, and Jenner concluded that the boy was immune to smallpox.

Initially this work was met with rejection, but he collected a few similar cases and published the results privately. In it he observed that the Latin word for cow is *vacca* and cowpox is *vaccinia*, and so named the new procedure *vaccination*.

Jenner conducted a nationwide survey in search of proof of resistance to smallpox among persons who previously had had cowpox. The results of this survey supported his theory and provided one of the world's first epidemiologic studies.

Henceforth, despite much controversy, vaccination spread rapidly in England, and by 1800 it had reached most European countries and made the jump to North America. Benjamin Waterhouse, a professor of physics at Harvard University introduced vaccination in New England, then persuaded Thomas Jefferson to let it be used in Virginia. Jefferson consented and made Waterhouse a vaccine agent in the National Vaccine Institute, an organization established to implement a national vaccination program in the United States. Gradually, vaccination replaced variolation, which was prohibited in England in 1840.

Jenner's work represents the first generally recognized scientific attempt to control an infectious disease by safe and effective immunization. Late in the 19th century, however, it became apparent that vaccination did not confer lifelong immunity and revaccination was necessary. Although mortality from smallpox had declined, recurrent epidemics showed that the disease was not fully controlled. Additional control measures were implemented in the 1950s, and smallpox was totally eradicated in most of Europe and North America.

The process of worldwide eradication was set in motion when the World Health Assembly received a report in 1958 of continued persistence of smallpox in sixty-three countries. In 1967, a global campaign began under the World Health Organization which finally eradicated smallpox in 1977.

Ignatz Semmelweis (1818–1865), the Father of Infection Control, was a Hungarian physician who demonstrated that *puerperal sepsis*, also known as childbed fever, was contagious and its incidence could be drastically reduced by hand washing.

While working in the Maternity Department of the Vienna Lying-in Hospital in 1847, Semmelweis realized that the number of cases of puerperal fever was much larger in one of his wards than the other. After testing a few hypotheses, he found that the number of cases was drastically reduced if doctors washed their hands carefully before examining a pregnant woman internally. The risk was particularly high if the physicians were in contact with corpses before they treated the women. Inasmuch as the germ theory of disease had not yet been developed, Semelweiss concluded that some unknown cadaveric material caused childbed fever.

Semmelweis lectured publicly about his results in 1850; however, the reception by the medical community was cold, if not hostile. Doctors were not eager to admit they may have caused many deaths, and Semmelweis's observations contradicted the current dogma which blamed diseases on an imbalance of basic "humours" in the body. Opponents also argued that even if his findings were correct, washing one's hands between patients would be too much work.

Semmelweis spent fourteen years lobbying for his ideas. He suffered a nervous breakdown in 1865 and was committed to an insane asylum where he soon died, ironically, from "blood poisoning," a blood-borne infection of the entire body.

The germ theory of disease was developed after Semmelweis's death, and he is now recognized as a pioneer of antiseptic policy, public health measures, and prevention of disease.

Louis Pasteur (1822–1895), the second Father of Microbiology (or Bacteriology), provided perhaps the greatest impetus to modern medical science that has ever been seen.[114] Pasteur was born in 1822, in Dole, France, into the family of a poor tanner, growing up in the town of Arbois. He gained degrees in Letters and in Mathematical Sciences before entering the École Normale Supérieure, an elite college. After serving briefly as professor of physics at Dijon Lycée in 1848, he became professor of chemistry at the University of Strasbourg, where he met and courted Marie Laurent, daughter of the university's rector, in 1849. They were married in that same year, and together had five children, only two of whom survived to adulthood; the other three died of typhoid. These personal tragedies inspired Pasteur to try to find cures for diseases such as typhoid. His early work involved important contributions in chemistry. In1854, he was named Dean of the new Faculty of Sciences in Lille. In 1856, he was made administrator and director of scientific studies of the <u>École Normale Supérieure</u>.

Beginning in the mid-1850s, Pasteur became interested in the fermentation of wine, observing that special microorganisms

---

[114] Geison GL, *The private science of Louis Pasteur.* Princeton University Press, Princton, NJ, 1995.

could account for the process and might also cause milk to turn sour and meat to decay. He demonstrated to the wine industry that if the product is heated to 60 Celsius (140 degrees Fahrenheit) for a short time, the growth of harmful bacteria was prevented and the wine would not go sour. Extending this theory, he proposed heating milk to a high temperature and pressure before bottling. The process that bears his name, *pasteurization*, is still used worldwide.

Pasteur's astute and careful observations allowed him to later connect bacteria with disease by demonstrating that silkworms could be killed by these tiny organisms. He devised a simple way to keep the worms disease free and rescued the French silk industry. This laid the foundation for *germ theory*, which stimulated a worldwide revolution in medical science.

The implications of Pasteur's work came to the attention of Edinburgh surgeon Lord **Joseph Lister** who, concerned about high post-operative mortality rates at his hospital, introduced disinfectant (antibacterial) sprays during operations, which prevented bacteria from entering a wound. He also introduced strict rules of hygiene to combat infections. The sterile methods developed drastically reduced the number of hospital deaths.

After his initial work, Pasteur became interested in disease prevention. He first turned his attention to anthrax, a serious bacterial disease of cattle, other animals, and humans. He effectively employed Jenner's concept and succeeded in producing a weakened and harmless culture of anthrax bacteria with which he inoculating cattle and sheep, inducing a mild form of the disease from which they recovered. When these animals were then put with others having a severe form of the disease they remained unaffected, indicating they were immune. Pasteur then extended his investigation to the virus that causes rabies, and developed an attenuated form of the virus that, when given by injection, prevents this disease.

Perhaps foremost among Pasteur's admirable qualities was the ability to survey all known data and evaluate all possible hypotheses. He experimented under strictly controlled conditions, and so when he obtained positive results, could point out the proper method for their application. About the discipline required to work in this fashion, he commented, "Imagination should give wings to our thoughts but we always need decisive experimental proof, and when the moment comes to draw conclusions and to interpret the gathered observations, imagination must be checked and documented by the factual results of the experiment." Pasteur is also often quoted for another famous remark: ."..dans les champs de l'observation, le hasard ne favorise que les esprits préparés" (In the field of observation, chance favors only the prepared mind.) Needless to say, these statements ring true to this day.

Pasteur became a national hero and was honored in many ways. He died at Saint-Cloud on 28 September 1895 and received a state funeral at the Cathedral of Notre Dame and his body placed in a permanent crypt at the Pasteur Institute that he founded and that continues to operate under his name. Regrettably, Semmelweis was not accorded similar honors until after his death.

Robert Koch (1843–1910),[115] the third Father of Microbiology (or Clinical Microbiology), was born in Germany and became interested in biology at an early age. He studied medicine at the University of Gottingen and was influenced by his renowned anatomy professor, Jacob Henle, who believed that living microscopic organisms caused infectious diseases.

After completing his medical studies in 1866, he became a district medical officer in Wollstein, Germany. During this time, he began to study anthrax and developed techniques allowing him to culture the causative bacillus. He demonstrated that the organism could not only be transmitted to other animals, but also could

---

[115] Brock TD, Robert *Koch: A Life in Medicine and Bacteriology.* ASM Press, Washingon, DC. (1999).

remain dormant for long periods in the form of spores (analogous to seeds), then return to its original disease-causing form when the proper conditions arose.

Koch did further important work on the study of diseases caused by bacterial infections of wounds, and provided a practical and scientific basis for controlling of such infections. He invented methods of culturing disease-causing bacteria in their pure form, which promoted better techniques for their identification and study. He developed four criteria designed to establish a causal relationship between a given microbe and a disease, commonly referred to as "Koch's postulates." Koch applied these postulates to establish the cause of anthrax and tuberculosis, but they were later generalized to other diseases. These criteria held sway in the medical world for many years, but have now been supplanted by modern techniques.

During his work, Koch discovered the bacteria that causes tuberculosis (*the tubercle bacillus*) and discovered the causative agent for cholera (*Vibrio cholerae*). He applied his knowledge of how these bacteria were transmitted to public health measures, such as personal hygiene and the proper treatment of water supplies. He also demonstrated that typhus, caused by a microbe (*Rickettsie prowazekii*), was spread from person to person through transmission by contact with body lice or fleas. He contributed to the work of others concerning the cause and treatment of malaria. Among many honors, he was awarded in 1905 the Nobel Prize for Physiology and Medicine.

Paul Ehrlich (1854–1915), the Father of Immunology and Chemotherapy, in a sense completed the work of Semmelweis, Pasteur and Koch by inventing a substance which, when placed into the body, could kill an infectious agent without killing the host.

Ehrlich was born in Upper Silesia, Germany, of Jewish parents. After receiving a medical degree in 1878, Ehrlich studied and developed techniques of using dyes to stain and identify various bodily tissues, blood cells, and bacteria.[116] The modern method of staining bacteria used today, the *gram stain*, is a result of his fundamental work. He also developed an effective method of staining and identifying the tubercle bacillus that Koch discovered. Koch, then Director the Berlin Institute for Infectious Diseases, appointed Ehrlich as one of his assistants, and Ehrlich began to study immunity and made important contributions to the field.

Ehrlich's work included evaluating chemicals that could go straight to the organisms at which they were aimed. Ehrlich called them "magic bullets." After working with numerous chemical agents, he began testing organic compounds containing arsenic and, after 606 trials, found arsphenamine, marketed as Salvarsan (later Neosalvarsan) and also known as "606." He demonstrated that this agent was effective against syphilis. At that time syphilis was a worldwide scourge, analogous to the AIDS of today, and this had motivated him to seek a cure. Ehrlich, like so many other discoverers before him, had to battle with much opposition before Neosalvarsan was finally accepted for the treatment of human syphilis. Ultimately the practical experience prevailed, and Ehrlich became famous as one of the main founders of modern chemotherapy. Among the numerous awards he received, he shared the highest scientific distinction, the Nobel Prize in 1908.

Ehrlich's insistence on the repeated and meticulous confirmation of the results of the many experiments he published, and the veneration and devotion shown to him by all his assistants, have been described by his former secretary, Martha Marquardt, whose biography of him has given us a personal picture of his life. As an interesting sidelight, in Frankfurt, Germany, the street in

---

[116] *Nobel Lectures*, Physiology or Medicine 1901-1921, Elsevier Publishing Company, Amsterdam, 1967.

which his Institute was situated was named Paul Ehrlichstrasse after him. Later, however, because of his Jewish identity and its related persecution, his name was removed. After the Second World War, however, when his birthplace, Strehlen, came under the jurisdiction of the Polish authorities, they renamed it Ehrlichstadt, in honor of its great son.

Ehrlich's life was depicted in the 1940 movie "Dr. Ehrlich's Magic Bullet," which focused on his search for a cure for syphilis. His character was portrayed by the actor, Edward G. Robinson. Interestingly, this film generated controversy because many thought the subject of syphilis too scandalous a topic for a motion picture in 1940. My, how times have changed. Another interesting tidbit is that this was the first recorded usage of the term "Magic Bullet."

Ehrlich became famous as one of the founders of modern chemotherapy, and was awarded the Nobel Prize for Medicine in 1908.

THE ONGOING AWAKENING OF SCIENTIFIC MEDICINE

"The most exciting phrase to hear in science, the one that heralds new discoveries, is not 'Eureka!' but 'That's funny'…"

Isaac Asimov

Although the most important triumphs in medicine during the nineteenth and early twentieth century concerned identification and prevention of infectious diseases, these and other advances spawned an awakening and appreciation of the strict rules of the scientific method. Following in this spirit, the subsequent number of important developments in scientific medicine has been nothing short of miraculous and too numerous to detail in a single volume such as this. These include the discovery and medical application of X-Rays in 1895 by a German, Wilhelm Roentgen, and the invention of the first practical electrocardiogram in 1906 by Willem Einthoven, a Dutchman. Both these individuals were awarded Nobel Prizes for their accomplishments. The many other advances such as development of immunization against polio and childhood diseases, the huge multiplicity of imaging techniques such as ultrasound and magnetic resonance, and various improvements in surgery and anesthesia, go on *ad infinitum*. My primary goal in this section, however, is to demonstrate how the relentless progression of scientific thought and methodology has gradually replaced the heretofore prevalent biases and myths, often based on intuition and apparent "logic." Unfortunately, many of these latter fallacies persist to this day, as I have detailed throughout this volume.

ADDITIONAL METHODS TO CONTROL INFECTIOUS DISEASES

After the causes, prevention, immunization and early chemical treatment for many bacterial and viral diseases were developed by the remarkable scientists noted above, the next major development—treatment through use of so-called antibiotics—was not forthcoming until the 1930s, presented in the sections below. But this discussion is best coupled with an exploration of the effects of the various medical advances on general humanity, especially during wars, periods in which impacts are quite profound and statistics resulting from successes and failures are relatively easily acquired.

The state of medicine in the United States, during the 1860s: During the American Civil War era and its early aftermath, just before the impact of Semmelweis, Pasteur and others, medical science was still primitive. While the average soldier believed the bullet offered the biggest risk, disease was actually the major killer. Of the Federal dead, roughly three of five died of disease, and of the Confederate troops, perhaps two of three. About half the deaths from infectious disease during the Civil War were caused by intestinal disorders, such as typhoid fever (which accounted for about one-quarter of noncombat deaths) and dysentery. The remainder died from pneumonia and tuberculosis. The camps themselves were laden with filth, fostering the rapid spread of bacterial and viral diseases among troops in close contact with one another. Epidemics of malaria spread through camps located next to stagnant swamps teeming with *anopheles* mosquito. Although treatment with quinine reduced fatalities, malaria nevertheless struck approximately one quarter of all servicemen; the Union army alone reported one million cases during the course of the war.

Lacking any means to deal with internal wounds involving the head, chest, and abdomen, surgeons were regularly forced to stand by helplessly while soldiers suffering these casualties were left to die. Significant wounds to the extremities usually resulted in the grisly practice of amputation. This was usually done to prevent infection from extending from an infected or gangrenous extremity. Since the bone saw (similar to the ordinary carpenter's saw) was used for this task, these practitioners were commonly referred to—ingloriously—as "sawbones," a now familiar moniker. Although the origin of this slang term is often tied to the Civil War, it actually had been attributed previously to Dickens in his 1837 novel *Pickwick Papers.* Fortunately for those subjected to this unpleasant procedure of amputation, pain was prevented through general anesthetics (chloroform and ether), already in use for several years. Most of the wounded received chloroform, the more convenient (although potentially more toxic) of the two. Opium and morphine were also generally available for pain control, but these drugs posed the additional risk of subsequent addiction, especially in those requiring their prolonged use.

This brief summary of medical experience during the Civil War era serves to underline how far medical science had yet to go before it could eventually reach its modern day successes.

After the civil war era, we learned from scientific experimentation about the underlying causes of diseases such as bacterial infections, and this resulted in the use of immunization and public health measures to prevent their occurrence and spread. But a whole new era was ushered in with early discoveries of additional chemical and biologic agents able to destroy bacteria. This began with the discovery of penicillin in 1929 by Alexander Fleming, a Scottish biologist and pharmacist. One day in 1928, before tossing some old bacterial culture dishes away, he noticed a blue-green mold growing on the culture of some harmful bacteria. The mold seemed to kill off the neighboring bacteria. A series of experiments later expanded his findings and led to the discovery of penicillin. This strain of *penicillia* could kill several kinds of harmful bacteria without damaging the human body. It was not until the late 1930s, however, that other scientists found a way to mass-produce penicillin, which then led to its production by British and American drug companies. Fleming received the Nobel Prize for Medicine in 1945. At that time he humbly said, "Nature makes penicillin; I just found it." But that comment must be tempered by what Pasteur had said decades previously, "Where observation is concerned, chance favors only the prepared mind." Fleming spent the rest of his career at St. Mary's Hospital in London until his death in 1955 of a heart attack.

The increasingly large production of penicillin allowed this agent to be used on a general clinical scale, especially during the Second World War and thereafter. This, plus the almost concomitant development of sulfa drugs, opened the floodgates to large list of additional antibiotics that continues expanding to this day. Shortly before the use of penicillin, however, the German firm, Bayer, in 1935 developed a chemical of the general class of "sulfa drugs." The initial member of the sulfa family, labeled Prontosil, was, together with penicillin, the first agents ever discovered that could effectively treat a range of bacterial infections inside the body, including streptococcal throat infections, blood infections and others. Penicillin proved to be very effective against the bacterial cause of syphilis, and, because of fewer side effects, quickly replaced the arsenical compounds developed by Ehrlich. Later Prontosil was further refined into its active molecule by the French at the Pasteur Institute into the active compound called sulfanilamide, the predecessor of a variety of similar drugs used to this day. As the first and only effective antibacterial agents available in the years before penicillin, sulfa drugs continued to thrive through the early years of World War II. They are credited with saving the lives of tens of thousands of patients including Franklin Delano Roosevelt, Jr. (son of President Franklin Delano Roosevelt) and Winston Churchill. These agents had a central role in preventing wound infections during the war. American soldiers were issued a first-aid kit containing sulfa pills and powder and were told to sprinkle it on any open wound.

After the antibiotic era began, accompanied by the introduction of other modern medical and surgical techniques during the Second World War, a dramatic reduction was noted in all infectious diseases. Moreover, during the Korean conflict, to employ modern medical treatment as early as possible after troops were wounded, mobile army surgical hospitals ("M.A.S.H." units) were created and placed in the field just behind combat zones beyond artillery range. Crucial lifesaving care was then brought to the wounded within minutes after an injury occurred.

The M.A.S.H. concept was first developed near the end of World War II, when they were initially called Echelon II hospital units. The M.A.S.H. units were fully mobile sixty bed truck-born units, amply staffed with medical and surgical personnel. They were later enlarged to one-hundred-fifty and then to two-hundred beds to accommodate the huge demand. They could be dissembled and moved within approximately six hours for rapid redeployment to other zones. During the prior half century, surgical care had advanced to the point that wounds could be approached and repaired in almost all parts of the body. The results were outstanding: The early treatment of the wounded, combined with a swift evacuation by helicopter to fixed facilities, helped lower the fatality rate to 2.5% from a previously recorded 4.5% during World War II. That meant if a soldier survived long enough to reach one of these units, his chances of living were 97.5%, a remarkable feat—especially when considering the dismal experience during the Civil War.

After Korea, M.A.S.H. units continued to serve in Vietnam, the 1991 Gulf War, and the conflicts in Iraq and Afghanistan in the 2000s. The huge success of this concept of trauma management through helicopter evacuation, use of paramedics, and advanced early application of surgical methods, infection control, and care of shock victims has been emulated in civilian city urban centers in the United States and throughout the world. Thus, notwithstanding the comedic movie and popular television series, these M.A.S.H units were serious vehicles that saved countless lives—a contribution that continues today. All these advances, and many others, again provide a tribute to scientific methods as applied to medicine.

ᑫᕐᑭ *Chapter Eighteen* ᕐᑕᑭ

EVIDENCE-BASED MEDICINE (EBM)

"Even if the open windows of science at first make us shiver after the cozy indoor warmth of traditional humanizing myths, in the end the fresh air brings vigor, and the great spaces have a splendor of their own."

Bertrand Russell

In contrast to alternative medicine, evidence-based medicine, or evidence-based practice, applies the best available evidence gained from the scientific method to clinical decision making, including medical and surgical treatments, laboratory and imaging tests, and many others. Regarding therapies, it seeks to assess the evidence of the risks and benefits of various treatments.

WHO IS A SCIENTIST?

We all commonly encounter statements that "scientists" have discovered something about almost anything. Upon exploring the issue further, we discover that we don't usually know who these scientists are. This raises the question of who is a scientist, and how s/he can be recognized as such. The answer is not as easy as one might imagine. A series of letters following one's name does not automatically confer the status of scientist. For instance, an MD or PhD after a name suggests that the basic qualifications are present, but we are all subject to biases and errors. Conversely, the absence of such degrees does not necessarily mean that one is not a scientist. Among other challenges, those working in scientific fields are often tempted to make unwarranted generalizations from anecdotal information. This constitutes perhaps the most serious and constant threat to scientific achievement, but erroneous conclusions can stem from faulty reasoning and misinterpretation of research reports. For instance, even though I possess an MD degree, I cannot conclude that a given treatment is effective if only flimsy or nonexistent research about it is available. However, we often encounter credentialed individuals who promote questionable conclusions or treatments, often, sadly, for financial gain. But how can an average individual avoid being seduced by such slick salesmen?

The most direct answer is that we should always be skeptical of any assertions that seem questionable or improbable, because spurious conclusions may seem probable to an untrained, uncritical person. When possible, try to determine the origin of such assertions, which may quickly expose the validity, weakness, or absence of underlying research. If you are unable or unqualified to evaluate this information, seek the opinions of recognized authorities qualified in the same scientific field. As Brian Dunning,[117] popular author and skeptical podcaster, aptly stated, "The fact that calling someone a scientist doesn't mean that he's smart, that he's right, that he thinks scientifically, or that he's anything more than a waste of space…All this means is that the label of 'scientist' is pretty darn worthless by itself."

ANIMAL RESEARCH

Since human research and medical advancement usually rely heavily on prior animal research, this issue must be addressed. As an unrepentant dog lover, I approach this topic with ambivalence. I am certainly sympathetic to our fellow primates, such as monkeys, but have far less affinity and sympathy for those lower in the animal kingdom, such as rodents, birds, insects (especially houseflies and fleas), reptiles, and progressing all the way down to bacteria (especially those that produce disease). Regardless of one's likes and dislikes, however, one point must be made clear beyond any doubt—animal experimentation is

---

[117] Dunning B. *Skeptoid: Critical Analysis of Pop Phenomena.* Thunderwood Press., 2007. p. 97.

absolutely indispensable to medical research, and it will remain so into the foreseeable future. Almost all of us owe our lives and comfort to past advances achieved in this way.

Although the practice dates back to ancient Greece, the need for animals in research has been obvious since the time of Pasteur, who confirmed the germ theory by inducing anthrax in sheep. Since then, animals have been used to test drug toxicity and efficacy before use in humans, assess the toxicology of potentially noxious agents, and help us to understand how and why certain diseases develop, among other critical tasks. Laboratory manipulation can now modify, remove, or replace specific genes to study disease; immunity and allergy can be studied and modified; and the information yielded will likely eliminate tissue rejection and allow for *xenotransplantation*, or the use of organs from other species to replace human ones. The best genetic models for human disease are provided by mice, but rats, pigs, sheep, fish, birds, and amphibians are also used. Despite the uproar provoked by various animal rights organizations attempting to force the discontinuation of animal testing in favor of computer methods or other means, the practice continues, and with good reason.

An example of the dividends provided by animal research is the discovery of insulin, the pancreatic hormone that controls blood sugar (glucose) levels. This hormone is produced in insufficient quantities in diabetics, which allows blood sugar levels to rocket up to levels that can prove fatal.

In 1921, while working in a laboratory with a group of dogs at the University of Toronto, Frederick Banting and Charles Best, working under Professor John MacLeod, observed that when the pancreas was removed, the dogs developed diabetes. They then extracted a substance from healthy canine pancreatic glands; when this substance was injected repeatedly into a diabetic dog, they noted that the blood sugar fell and the animal became outwardly healthy and regained lost strength. After this initial success, they named their substance insulin, developed methods for its purification, and then turned to cattle to obtain a larger supply.

In January 1922, they tested insulin on a fourteen-year-old boy who suffered from diabetes so severe he was near death. After repeated injections, the boy rapidly regained strength and vitality, no longer experiencing symptoms attributable to high blood sugar. They continued testing other diabetic volunteers, obtained the same results, and the rest is history. In 1923, the Toronto team received the Nobel Prize in Physiology/Medicine. Since that breakthrough, insulin has saved millions of lives, and continues to benefit humans, as well as diabetic animals. Although that advance occurred long ago, the use of animals for research remains just as important, if not more so, for the welfare of almost all creatures on the planet. No matter how sophisticated computer modeling or other technologies can be, they are unlikely to replace animal experimentation.

The information derived from animal testing is critical for the advancement of medical science. The use of animals, particularly dogs and cats, should be limited to urgent necessities, and all animal research must be conducted responsibly to minimize the pain and suffering of the subjects, and avoided entirely when alternative methods are available. In most parts of the world, medical agencies have teamed with governmental overseers to provide a humane and sensible means to conduct such research. Hopefully efforts by obstructionist groups will not impede future advances that will benefit humans and many of our other fellow species.

HUMAN RESEARCH

After studies in animals have established the likely safety of a proposed new treatment, often a drug, preliminary studies in volunteer humans further establish safety and efficacy. After passing this hurdle, larger double-blind, placebo-controlled clinical trials that represent the most widely accepted form of testing new drugs can be undertaken. This type of research, however, is not always available or possible, such as in the application of new surgical techniques. Alternative research designs are occasionally used, although they are often less conclusive. For instance, *historical controls*— data taken from earlier observations—are occasionally used to compare with results of a new treatment. *Case control designs* seek out persons who have suffered from a certain disease and compare them with a matched group free of this disease. Antecedent factors that might identify a cause for the disease in question are investigated.

Most medical research involves study extending far beyond controlled trials. This includes observations from laboratories or clinics to learn about efficacy of laboratory or diagnostic tests, disease causation and progress, testing of hypotheses, etc. Other aspects of health care fall even further outside the realm of strict scientific study, such as quality and value of life judgments; nevertheless, the scientific approach seeks, through careful observation, to apply effective methods to diagnosis, treatment, and predictions of outcome in many circumstances.

Almost all current studies employ statistical methods with the aim of establishing true, or *statistically significant*, relationships or differences, as opposed to random variations. To facilitate the publication, transmission, and sharing of research results, a huge number of medical and scientific journals are now available. Almost all these publications employ the *peer review process*, in which recognized authorities, or *referees*, in the same field critically evaluate each submitted manuscript to determine suitability for publication. The final decision is generally the responsibility of the journal's editor-in-chief, who is usually a recognized authority in the same general field. Although far from perfect, this system seems to be fairly effective, though not foolproof; there are occasional incidences of biases and outright fraud. Moreover, because peer reviewers are human, they are subject to the same biases that afflict all of us. Their criticism and recommendations for publication have been shown to be subject to biases based on their own preexisting beliefs.[118]. Having been involved in this process for many years, I have observed numerous instances of this type of bias. Often the opinions of the two reviewers differ dramatically, whereupon the editor must render a final decision or request additional opinions.

More insidious forms of bias may also confound an issue. A research finding is less likely to be true when studies contain relatively small numbers of subjects, when the measured effects are smaller, when a tested population fails to match all characteristics of the population to which the results are to be applied, and when there is greater financial and other interest producing prejudice. For many current scientific fields, claimed research findings may often be simply accurate measures of a prevailing bias. [119]

MISTAKES IN SCIENTIFIC RESEARCH

As the volume of published medical research expands, so too does the frequency of reported errors. According to a recent review in the August 11, 2011 issue of the *Wall Street Journal*, the number of studies published in research journals has risen 44% since 2001, but the number retracted due to inaccuracy has increased fifteen-fold in the same period.

In an attempt to determine whether these retractions were due to simple error or outright fraud, RG Steen[120] reviewed 788

---

[118] Mahoney MJ. *Publication prejudices: An experimental study of confirmatory bias in the peer review system.* Cognitive Therapy and Research. 1977;1:161-175.
[119] Ioannidis J.P.A. *Why Most Published Research Findings Are False* PLoS Med. 2005 August; 2(8): e124.

[120] Steen, RG. *Misinformation in the medical literature: what role do error and fraud play?* J Med Ethics. .2010.038125.

retracted studies involving medicine and other sciences, including biology, chemistry, pharmacology, physics, and others. He estimated that about 74% of these were retracted because of simple errors, and 26% due to fraud. What is even more disconcerting is that authors with a prior record of fraud were frequently guilty of repetitive violations. The delay between initial publication and subsequent retraction has also been steadily rising, from 5.25 months in 2000 to 31.6 months in 2009. This lengthy delay is hazardous to those trying to use the information to manage patients or to develop hypotheses for further study. Unfortunately, most scientific institutions and journals lack the resources to investigate misconduct properly, let alone ferret out errors in data acquisition and analysis. Fortunately, scientific methods almost always rely on duplication of results in other centers and verification through alternative means. Thus, while science is not perfect, it is eventually self-correcting.

An additional, little-known problem, called *publication bias*, often compounds this issue. Medical journals are generally disproportionately prone to accepting positive results when presented with a new concept or treatment. Editors may be less critical in their evaluations because of the seductive nature of a new concept that seems, at least on the surface, logical. Also, aspiring researchers often wish to present positive results, because they enhance their scientific status which, in turn, increases their chances of tenure, promotion or fame. Additionally, pressure to publish creates potential biases toward conscious or unconscious manipulation of the results in a positive direction. Minor infractions of this type seldom trigger retractions, but probably distort results to some degree.

After initial positive results are published, subsequent research usually confirms or refutes the findings. If later study results in disagreement, the negative findings are readily accepted for publication, but this may not occur for months or years. However, negative findings would seldom be considered as an initial offering by a standard journal; they are not as appealing as positive results. Not only does publication bias create a disproportionately high incidence of positive results, but they are often picked up in the general media and touted as major breakthroughs. This often leads to a misinterpretation about the cause of a given disease, or to inflated hopes that successful treatment is imminent. Unfortunately, the failure of initial hope— as determined by later research—often never reaches these same publications, and the false hopes or expectations persist.

What can unsuspecting physicians and the public do to protect themselves from misleading and potentially dangerous erroneous information? Publication of retractions does help, at least by encouraging honest researchers to be more careful in future studies. Opposing results that refute the erroneous reports may allow for skepticism in less time than publication of a retraction. But, perhaps most importantly, the medical profession and general public must be highly skeptical of initial reports claiming miraculous successes or breakthroughs. This pertains to almost all information about health. When studies first go public, the best policy is to wait sufficiently long to allow confirmation by other research.

The huge and constant proliferation of medical research eventually reaches its final and most important destination—the individual medical practitioner—who is then responsible for its incorporation into practice. To function effectively, the practitioner must continually evaluate published reports, the scientific strength of various studies, and apply this information to the daily care of patients. For instance, since information derived from epidemiologic studies is considered less than ideal, it may or may not provide a satisfactory basis for managing or advising patients. The relationship between alcohol consumption and cardiovascular disease is a good example, for numerous epidemiologic studies have clearly established that the consumption of one or two ounces of alcohol daily is associated with a lower incidence of cardiovascular mortality when compared to non-drinkers.[121] Since prospective controlled studies have not been performed to gain more conclusive information about this apparent cause-and-effect relationship, should the practitioner advise a teetotaler to begin drinking? This presents a real dilemma, for a physician cannot guarantee that such a lifestyle change will reduce health risk. Moreover, lobbying for alcohol consumption poses the danger of inducing some individuals to begin drinking heavily, which could in turn result in overconsumption, or even addiction. Thus most practitioners approve of the continuation of modest alcohol consumption but generally do not urge non-drinkers to begin imbibing.

Burdened by so much information, individual practitioners are regularly assisted by numerous guidelines from virtually all the medical specialties. They are produced by panels of recognized experts in their respective fields, and cover a wide variety of issues related to medical practice. Guidelines generally include the level of research strength available for the support of each recommendation, and advice against methods or procedures that are considered useless or dangerous.

We must bear in mind that EBM is still in its infancy—barely over fifty-years old, with the term coined in 1990. Although this term is new, evidence—evolving gradually over the past century—has guided medical practice for a lengthy period. Individual practice is based on myriad factors, including background scientific education and information gained from medical journals and conferences. Experience gained from repetitive individual observations (clinical acumen) plays a major role.

While the modern physician attempts to incorporate tenets derived from guidelines, they often do not cover all possible

---

[121] Rimm E. *Alcohol and cardiovascular disease*. Current Atherosclerosis Reports. 2000; 2:529-535.

scenarios. Thus physicians continue to exercise their best judgment, relying on traditional principles as well as the most recent evidence. In actual practice, medical practice involves a combination of clinical expertise (clinical acumen), research evidence, and patients' preferences.[122]

BIAS FAVORING THE USE OF NEW DRUGS

We have all enjoyed the fruits of research sponsored and performed by pharmaceutical companies. Their efforts have enriched and prolonged our lives through major advances in the prevention and control of many serious diseases. For all this, and for the many inevitable future advances, we owe the industry a debt of gratitude.

However, anyone who watches TV can't avoid the almost constant bombardment of pharmaceutical ads, touting the virtues of each drug offering, until you receive a litany of side effects and other cautions. All of these are brand-name drugs, most of which are currently operating under patent protection—meaning that, until the patent expires, no other producer can market the same product. The illusion these products are inherently superior is, to some extent, a result of the availability bias—they are constantly thrust into our consciousness. Also we are led to believe that price relates directly to quality. With regard to this latter issue, we are all, doctors and patients, regularly shocked by the hefty price of these drugs. This triggers a natural curiosity about the justification for these charges, which often reach several dollars per dose. What's even more important to most of us, however, is how we can reduce or avoid such burdensome expenses. So let's explore these issues and, hopefully, save some money.

We first need to look at the financial incentives within the pharmaceutical industry. Although estimates range widely, drug

---

[122] Haynes RB, Devereaux, PJ, and Guyatt, GH. Clinical expertise in the era of evidence-based medicine and patient choice. Evid Based Med 2002;7:36-38.

development is a very expensive proposition. Each successful new drug costs, on average, roughly $800 million to develop and, depending on many variables, this number can reach $1.5 billion. Why so expensive?

First, the process begins with exploring a number of molecular compounds that offer promise, progressing into early testing for safety in animals and eventually to volunteer humans. False starts along the way increase expenses without producing viable products. After early testing appears promising for a given drug, then large, double-blind trials are undertaken before the FDA grants final approval. Although the original patents for each successful product last for twenty years, they are obtained before clinical trials begin, so the effective life of a drug patent is between seven and twelve years, meaning the time a drug can be sold under patent protection is often significantly limited. Although each pill is manufactured at a miniscule cost, great sums of money must be recouped in a short time to yield any financial gain. This leads to decoupling immediate costs and individual drug pricing. Although average profits within the pharmaceutical industry are attractive, they are probably not excessive considering the substantial risks.

Given the dynamics of drug production, I can understand the industry's position, but feel compelled to enter the discussion on the side of the consumer. In many ways he/she is in a situation similar to going against the house in a casino—as we know, the odds are on the house's side. Since all advertised products are brand-named, they are usually patent protected and inevitably very expensive. They are also all relatively new; however, being new does not automatically confer better results.

I object to advertising prescription-only drugs to the public for two reasons. First, the cost of advertising inevitably forces prices higher. Second, patients pressure physicians to prescribe these expensive products. Since many patients have insurance to cover the purchase of these big-ticket products, physicians often find it easier to comply with patient requests, and the effort to seek cheaper alternatives is discouraged, even when they may be just as effective. Notwithstanding corporations' First Amendment rights, this principle is wrong.

Aggressive marketing is persuading many people to overpay for medication. According to IMS Health, a pharmaceutical intelligence company which tracks drug sales and marketing, drug makers spent $4.3 billion to reach consumers and $6.6 billion on promotions aimed at physicians. These tactics seem to be succeeding. *Consumer Reports* states that, in a recent poll, 20% of respondents said they asked for a drug they'd learned about from advertising, and 59% of those said their doctor agreed to write a prescription for that product. Compounding this problem is that, at least when it comes to pain relief, higher-priced medications produce stronger placebo responses than those that are thought to be cheaper. This conclusion is based on a study[123] in which two groups of volunteers received identical placebo pills ostensibly designed to reduce pain. The first group was told the cost of each pill was $2.50; the second group, 10¢. In response to painful stimuli, the group recciving what they thought was the expensive medication experienced significantly more relief than those receiving the cheaper one. These results not only support the power of the placebo effect, but also help to feed the coffers of the pharmaceutical companies.

The influence of the pharmaceutical industry extends further and more covertly, and this is especially troubling.[124] Concerned by bias and falsehoods creeping into pharmaceutical promotions, in 1981 the FDA established standards for all medication ads, mandating they must consist of "true statements relating to side effects, contraindications, and effectiveness." This

---

[123] Waber RL, Shiv B, Carmon Z, and Ariely D. *Commercial features of placebo and therapeutic efficacy.* JAMA 2008; 299:1016-7.

[124] Washington HA, *Flacking for Big Pharma*, American Scholar, 2011; 80:22-34.

was supposed to present a "fair balance" of statements about medication risks and benefits. But how accurately has this standard been followed?

In 1991, the editors of the *Annals of Internal Medicine,* a well-respected journal, studied a large number of their own ads. This study, which included a careful analysis by independent reviewers of the references cited by those ads, demonstrated that 57% had no educational value, 40% failed the fair-balance test, and 44% contained information that could result in improper prescribing. Overall, their reviewers would have recommended against publishing of 28% of the advertisements. Subsequently, the FDA issued eighty-eight letters accusing drug companies of advertising violations between 1997 and 2002. This caused advertising revenue to the *Annals of Internal Medicine* from drug companies to fall by $1.5 million, which resulted in the departure of the editorial staff. At the time of the exodus, Robert Fletcher, the journal's co-editor, stated that "The pharmaceutical industry showed us that the advertising dollar could be a two-edged sword, a carrot or a stick. If you ever wondered whether they play hardball, that was a pretty good demonstration that they do." Unfortunately, no evidence has surfaced since then to show that this situation has improved.

The shenanigans of large pharmaceutical companies do not stop here. We have recently discovered another unethical, but not illegal, activity some of these companies employ—the *seeding trial.*[125] This term applies to research studies involving a drug that has already been approved for general use, which are often called *phase-4 trials.* Although ostensibly for research purposes, these trials are marketing ploys masquerading as scientific studies. The company—often its marketing arm—recruits numerous practicing physicians to serve as investigators, who are in turn paid to recruit

---

[125] Krumholz SD, Egilman DS and Ross JS. *Study of neurontin: Titrate to effect, profile of safety (STEPS) trial.* Arch. Int. Med. 171; 2011:1100-1107.

patients to serve as study subjects. The companies' primary goal is to expose physicians to a new drug and have them interact with the company sponsors and its sales representatives in order to influence prescribing patterns. In reality, however, the investigators are the research subjects. They are charged with recording the efficacy and tolerability of a given drug at various dosage levels and conveying the data to the company or its representative. These studies are not blinded or controlled, and the data obtained are imprecise at best. Results may be published although, given their poor design, journal referees are likely to recommend against it. The company benefits in two ways. First, the physician investigators become familiar with the drug and so are more likely to prescribe it after the study is completed. Second, this also serves to discourage use of competitive products. Because of their vague nature and lack of transparency, these projects may be difficult to recognize by outside authorities, and even more difficult to limit. Because of these factors, the extent of these practices is largely unknown. Since the drugs have already been released for general use and the studies are not illegal, they are beyond the FDA's jurisdiction. The *institutional review boards* (IRBs) of medical facilities are supposed to scrutinize such studies for compliance with accepted research standards, but the members may also be misled, or may be personally involved—a conflict of interest.

Physicians and IRB members are being made aware of the nature of these phase-4 trials through medical publications. Patients are cautioned about participation in research involving recently approved drugs, although they are generally not subjected to undue risk. They will also be alerted by the need to sign consent forms for research participation, which is mandated by the IRB that evaluated the protocol. Publications exposing this practice will hopefully discourage further misleading activities by the companies.

For the most part, medical journals are overly dependent on pharmaceutical advertising, which can provide a major portion of their operating revenues. This allows drug companies to significantly influence them. Companies may insist that their products receive only favorable editorial reviews, and that the journal publishes only positive research results.

Of greater concern is the fact that these companies can pervert the content of research studies in various ways. These include comparing a drug against a competitor's drug in the wrong strength, prematurely stopping a trial, testing in very small groups, and engaging in *data mining*, a form of cherry picking, in which a study is scrutinized to find small groups that apparently benefit from given drug—a well-known statistical aberration. Although probably rare, primary data can be distorted unless subjected to the scrutiny of a disinterested outside party or the prospective medical journal itself, and these are practices not usually employed. Finally, as already noted, bias is easily tilted toward the publication of only positive results, while negative findings languish, with or without pressure from the pharmaceutical companies.

Most physicians understand the considerable limitations of pharmaceutical advertising, paying little attention to ads in journals and even less to those in the media. Nevertheless, we cannot control covert interference or data manipulation before publication that encourages sales of the most expensive drugs. Our main defense against these tactics is to carefully analyze available data and compare the high-priced, patented, brand-name products to generic alternatives.

Knowledge of the problems relative to drug research is important, and physicians as well as the public must be critical of new treatments, always comparing them with older, generic forms that are equally effective or even better. Disallowing advertising in journals would be helpful, but is impractical. Open-access journals, including Public Library of Science publications that reject advertising and are freely available online, would also benefit the system greatly. Books such as Angell's *The Truth about the Drug Companies*, and Abramson's *Overdosed America*, are reliable sources for detecting industrial improprieties.

The unethical practices of pharmaceutical companies are reflected in the increasing numbers of fraud and abuse cases resulting in federal financial recoveries between 1996 and 2010.[126] According to reports involving the Federal False Claims Act, fraud recoveries of $5 million and higher totaled $3.9 billion between 2001 and 2005, and rose to a staggering $8.1 billion between 2006 and 2010. Whistleblowers from within the companies triggered the vast majority of these actions. Reasons for these settlements include fraudulent and off-label marketing, misbranding, kickbacks, fraudulent pricing, and the selling of contaminated drugs. Virtually all the major companies have been involved in one or more settlements—a sorry testimonial to financial greed. But the stakes are high. Prescription drug spending in the United States increased from $40 billion in 1990 to $234 billion in 2008, and now accounts for about 10% of health care expenditures. In comparison with total revenues, fraud and abuse settlements must seem minor to pharmaceutical giants.

What about generic drugs? They are uniformly cheaper, but to what extent can these be substituted for brand-name products? Generally, if the same drug exists in both forms, it is OK to opt for the cheaper, generic version. All generic drugs are required to have the same active ingredient, strength, dosage form, and route of administration as brand name, or *reference*, product. The FDA assures the generic product will perform as does its respective brand name equivalent through the review of bioequivalence data. This standard applies to all generic drugs. For the best advice on this subject, see *Consumer Reports* Best Buy Drugs, which

---

[126] Qureshi ZP, Sartor OS, Xirasagar S, et al. *Pharmaceutical Fraud and Abuse in the United States,* 1996-2010. Arch. Int. Med. 2011; 171:1503-1506.

covers 25 classes of drugs for more than 35 conditions. It is available online at http://www.consumerreports.org/health/best-buy-drugs/index.htm.

In some instances, a single category of drugs contains both branded and generic versions with similar effects; those that are older are the generics. These latter forms are usually equally effective, but far cheaper. Examples in this category include, among others, several statin drugs such as simvastatin, or Zocor, used for lowering cholesterol levels, and several drugs for controlling blood pressure and blood sugar levels. In some instances, the branded drugs may be more powerful, but if the desired result can be obtained with the generic version, use the latter.

There are several other instances of functional overlap between old and new drugs despite differences in their chemical structures. Their chemical composition may be altered to market them as a new drug, and then they are often considered as "me too" drugs that exist primarily to provide the company with income. One of these is Avodart (dutasteride), used to control enlargement of the prostate gland (BPH). The retail price for this drug is around $4.30 a day as compared to a slightly different generic, finasteride, which affects the prostate gland in the same way and costs approximately 48¢ a day. My advice to the consumer before embarking on a new and expensive product is to consult your physician about possible older—but equally effective—generic products.

In summary then, since there are numerous ways to reduce drug costs, I strongly advise the readers to consult with their physicians to explore possibilities for substitutions and alternatives. Above all, do not insist on obtaining the most expensive product, even though you have seen it on television.

There are always safety issues attached to using newly approved drugs. After initial release into the marketplace, new drugs may be in general use for lengthy periods before side-effects become apparent. The gravity of these undesirable effects may be serious enough to mandate a drug's withdrawal from the market. A good example is Vioxx (rofecoxib).

In 1999, the FDA granted the Merck Co. approval to begin marketing a new drug, Vioxx (rofecoxib) for use in general pain control, including that resulting from certain types of arthritis and from menstrual periods. This drug belongs to a class called *COX-2 inhibitors*, which are similar to non-steroidal anti-inflammatory drugs, or NSAIDS, such as ibuprofen (Advil). Vioxx joined the newly-released Celebrex (celecoxib) as a breakthrough in low risk pain management. The new agents allegedly caused fewer gastrointestinal side effects (ulcers and inflammation) than their older counterparts and, despite lack of evidence, claimed they also had superior pain-killing properties. Later studies have refuted these latter claims, which were probably attributable to the placebo effect, which was, in turn, probably linked to their high price.

Three years after its introduction, data began accumulating that Vioxx was associated with an elevated rate of heart attacks and strokes. This drug's undesirable effects probably resulted from the promotion of blood clotting in the arteries supplying the heart and brain. As information continued to mount, Merck withdrew Vioxx from the market on Sept. 30, 2004. By then, at least eighty-million people worldwide had taken it. FDA analysts estimated that in the five years the drug was on the market, Vioxx caused between 88,000 and 139,000 heart attacks, 30% to 40% of which were probably fatal. Similar unfavorable effects were found for Pfizer's Bextra (valdecoxib). This drug was introduced in 2001 and withdrawn in 2005. Although Celebrex is still marketed, it also has been associated with increased cardiovascular events –fewer than the withdrawn drugs, but not free of them

Although the older NSAIDs are suspected of increasing the risk of cardiovascular events to a lesser extent, at least one, naproxen, seems to be fairly safe in this regard. Moreover, in compared with the newer COX-2 agents, these older drugs seem to cause no greater gastrointestinal side effects when taken together with antacid drugs such as Prilosec (omeprazole). Given these factors, coupled with the fact that pain-relieving powers between the drug classes are equal, there is little justification for the use of the newer agents under any circumstance.

So, what lessons can the public and physicians learn from these examples? As noted, always attempt to find older, generic drugs that have been in use for a long period of time. A longer track record provides greater assurance of safety. And the same caveat applies to the cost of drugs—more expensive does not mean better. Unless the reasons for their use is compelling, avoid the newest drugs until they have been in use for at least two to three years and, if possible, for a period of five to ten years.[127]

LOW HANGING FRUIT: DRUG TREATMENT OF PSYCHIATRIC ILLNESS

Mental problems are an especially enticing target for pharmaceutical companies. The diagnosis of emotional illnesses of all types is constantly changing, owing partially to the fact that defining these maladies is subjective and not amenable to laboratory testing. Thus the criteria for diagnoses are established by panels of experts, and are based on consensus and not by anything resembling hard data. Even minor mental quirks are now often classed as illness and, therefore, likely to invite treatment. Various degrees of anxiety—with or without depression—are the most prevalent of these disorders. The most recent version of the *Diagnostic and Statistical Manual of Mental Disorders, 4th Edition (DSM-IV-TR),* published by the American Psychiatric Association (APA), includes all currently recognized mental health disorders, listing a staggering 365 diagnoses. According to the

---

[127] Schiff GD, Galanter WD, Duhig J, et al. *Principles of conservative prescribing.* Arch. Intern. Med. 2011; 171:1433-40.

National Institute of Mental Health, 26% of all individuals in the U.S.A. will suffer from some type of mental illness in any given year. Anxiety disorders involve 18% of our population, and major depressive disorders, 6.7%. A large survey of randomly selected adults from our population, sponsored by the National Institute of Mental Health (NIMH) and conducted between 2001 and 2003, revealed that 46 percent met criteria for at least one mental illness within four broad categories at some time in their lives. The "anxiety disorders," included phobias and post-traumatic stress disorder (PTSD); "mood disorders," including major depression and bipolar disorders; "impulse-control disorders," including various behavioral problems and attention-deficit/hyperactivity disorder (ADHD); and "substance use disorders." Strikingly, of those affected within the previous year, a third were receiving drug treatment—up from a fifth in a similar survey ten years earlier

Historically, treatment of many emotional problems was accomplished by verbal interaction with therapists (psychotherapy), sometimes referred to as the "Freudian approach." Inasmuch as more potent drugs were unavailable, this management might include mild tranquilizers (sedatives) such as phenobarbital. With the discovery of so-called "psychoactive" drugs beginning in the late 1950s, the idea that mental disorders arose from various types of "chemical imbalances" in the brain became fashionable. This highly tenuous hypothesis has never been validated.[128] Nevertheless, the concept of an underlying tangible brain disorder has provided a rationale for the development and use of many drugs to combat these presumed "chemical imbalances." It also destigmatizes the emotional disorders, allowing patients to blame a physical malady rather than dreaded abnormalities of emotions that could presumably be willfully controlled.

---

[128] Angell M. The Epidemic of Mental Illness: Why? *New York Review of Books*, June 23, 2011, and The Illusions of Psychiatry, *New York Review of Books*, July 14, 2011.

Strong economic forces have further promoted the aggressive use of expensive drugs for the following reasons: First, psychotherapy performed by psychiatrists is time consuming and thus not well compensated. It is more cost-efficient for these physicians simply to establish diagnoses of mental disorders and become "pill-pushers." The more time-consuming "one-on-one" sessions, if performed at all, could then be relegated to psychologists, social workers, and other therapists. Second, the pharmaceutical industry has been more than eager to promote drug use, and, in the process, subsidize the psychiatric profession directly and indirectly, i.e., showering them with gifts and free drug samples, hiring them as "key opinion leaders" (consultants and speakers), subsidizing conferences, meals, etc. Not surprisingly, psychiatrics receive more financial support than any other medical specialty.[129]

A wholesale shift to drug therapy requires strong evidence of its efficacy, meaning that the psychoactive drugs must be shown to be superior to placebos or other treatment modes. But how much do we know about the use of these drugs in the light of competing approaches?

With regard to antidepressants, Kirsch[130] has presented convincing evidence that they are no better than placebos, at least in the long run. His conclusion was derived from a fifteen-year study. Initially he reviewed thirty-eight published clinical trials that evaluated treatments for depression, including placebos, psychotherapy and no treatment. Most trials lasted for six to eight weeks, and during that time, patients tend to improve somewhat even without treatment. Kirsch found that placebos were three times more effective than no treatment and only minimally inferior to the "active" drugs. After such equivocal results, he reviewed

[129] Carlat D. Unhinged: The Trouble with Psychiatry-a Doctor's revelations about a Profession in Crisis, Free Press, New York, 2010. p.111.
[130] Kirsch I. *The Emperor's New Drugs: Exploding the Antidepressant Myth*, Basic Books, New York, 2011.

information obtained from the US Food and Drug Administration (FDA). This includes all studies—published and unpublished—evaluating a given drug. If the results of placebo-controlled studies show the effectiveness of a new drug in two trials or more, the drug is generally approved, even if it fails to show improvement in multiple other studies. After including unpublished information, Kirsch concluded that there was no convincing evidence that this class of drugs was more effective than placebos, at least in the long term. This included the older drugs, the so-called "tricyclic" class. e.g. Elavil[R] (Amitriptyline) and the newer "selective serotonin reuptake inhibitors (SSRIs), exemplified by Prozac (fluoxetine), Celexa. (citalopram), Lexapro (escitalopram), Zoloft (sertraline), Paxil (paroxetine), and others. Kirsch was struck by another unexpected finding: In his earlier study and in work by others, he observed that even treatments not considered antidepressants—including synthetic thyroid hormone, opiates, sedatives, stimulants, and some herbal remedies such as St. John's wort—were as effective as antidepressants in alleviating the symptoms of depression.

Even more interesting, Kirsch encountered another confounding influence, the so-called "enhanced placebo" effect, which can cause the active agent under study to appear disproportionately effective. Although double-blinded trials are designed to eliminate bias on the part of those providing and receiving the experimental medicines, this may not always be the case. Potential side-effects of the active medicines are explained to the subjects prior to the studies. When these effects are encountered, subjects are more apt to conclude they are receiving the active drug rather than the placebo, thus encouraging the belief that they are more likely to gain better results, and this provides a boost toward favoring the new drug. Since most new drugs produce more side effects than do placebos, this paradoxically skews the results toward producing more beneficial placebo effects in the groups experiencing side effects. This sounds counterintuitive, but the conclusion seems warranted. Kirsch suggests further that the reason antidepressants appear to work better in relieving severe depression than in less severe cases is that severely depressed patients are likely to be on higher doses and therefore experience more side effects. To investigate whether side effects bias responses, Kirsch reviewed trials that employed "active" placebos instead of inert ones. An active placebo is one that itself generates side effects, such as atropine—a drug that, among other things, produces a noticeably dry mouth. In trials using atropine as the placebo, there was no difference between the antidepressant and the active placebo. Despite observations of this type, however, the overall weight of evidence seems to support the beneficial effect of antidepressant drugs at least for those individuals suffering from the most severe forms of depression.[131]

For obvious reasons, drug companies vigorously champion publication of positive studies in medical journals and strive to have doctors know about them, while the negative ones remain buried in the FDA archives. This practice greatly biases the medical literature, medical education, and treatment decisions.

How well do non-pharmacological approaches to mental illnesses stack up against drugs? Surprisingly well. Whitaker,[132] in an overview of medications for all types of mental disorders, presents evidence that psychotherapy—now commonly called "cognitive behavioral therapy"—is as effective as, or better than, drugs in treating both depression and the common psychotic disorder, schizophrenia—at least long term. This approach also avoids the bothersome side effects of drugs. He also presents evidence that drugs may even be detrimental in the long-term management of various anxiety disorders.

---

[131] Fournier JC, DeRubeis RJ, Hollon SD, et al. Antidepressant drug effects and depression severity: a patient-level meta-analysis. JAMA 2010;303:47-53.

[132] Whitaker R. Anatomy of an Epidemic: Magic Bullets, Psychiatric Drugs, and the Astonishing Rise of Mental Illness in America, Crown Publishers, New York, N.Y., 2010, pp. 336-347.

Although not well understood, exercise also may be quite useful in combating depression. Both Whitaker and Kirsch have presented convincing evidence that this form of treatment for this disorder is just as effective as drugs, and is now an accepted form of treatment in the U.K. Moreover, the antidepressant benefits of exercise seem to increase over time. Twenty minutes of exercise three days a week seems to be enough to produce the antidepressant effect, and the kind of exercise that is practiced does not seem to matter much. Walking and running are equally effective, and anaerobic exercise like weight training is as effective as aerobic exercise. Epidemiological studies indicate that exercise can prevent depression as well as ameliorate it.[133] Adding a personal note, I can provide some support for the emotional benefits of this treatment mode. For many years I have directed our local cardiac rehabilitation program, which includes those suffering from heart disorders of almost all types. The program consists primarily of regular exercise conditioning, and—although admittedly anecdotal—I receive regular feedback from patients saying that they are less depressed and experience a better overall sense of well-being after several weeks of exercise conditioning. Adding to its advantages, exercise carries little risk of side effects and clearly has benefits extending far beyond combating emotional problems.

TESTOSTERONE: ANOTHER PHARMACEUTICAL PLUM

Testosterone is the normal male hormone, manufactured by the testicles, that accounts for masculine features such as muscle size and strength, facial hair, sexual performance, and many others. In recent months, flurries of advertisements have appeared that sound something like this: "Fatigued, low energy, depressed mood, low sex drive. Could it be that your body's testosterone is too low,

---

[133] Strawbridge WJ, Deleger S, Roberts RE, Kaplan GA. Physical activity reduces risk of subsequentdepression for older adults. Am J Epidemiol 2002; 156:328-34.

also known as low T?" The ads go on to say that as some men grow old, their testosterone levels decline, recommending that they consult their physicians about testosterone replacement therapy. Simultaneously, other targeted medical ads to physicians issue a plea for the general screening of patients for blood levels of testosterone. They imply that low levels could explain those symptoms noted above and that relief may result from administered testosterone, usually applied with a patch on the skin—predictably quite expensive. But these symptoms are common in all aging individuals—male or female, and unrelated to the presence or absence of testosterone. Compounding this problem, testosterone output in males normally falls with age, so these levels in the bloodstream decline an average about 1.2 percent a year after the age of forty. Normal testosterone levels usually refer to what is found in normal men in their twenties. But even the definition of normal for younger men can be misleading, for these levels can vary markedly over the course of a day. Even in healthy men in their twenties, at some time during the day, up to 15% of them have testosterone levels up to 50% or more below their presumed normal levels.[134] Obviously, a greater percentage of men beyond the age of sixty will test below this range.

Although the FDA has approved the use of testosterone specifically for those individuals with severe physical hormonal deficiencies involving the testicles, the floodgates are open for unwitting physicians and eager patients to use this hormone in an "off label" fashion, aimed at a substantial portion of the forty million men in the U.S. over the age of fifty. This provides a great opportunity for the pharmaceutical industry to "medicalize" the normal process of aging.

Given the uncertainties noted above, how does the individual determine if he is really deficient in testosterone? The

---

[134] Groopman J. *How Doctors Think.* p. 209, Houghton Mifflen Co. New York, N.Y. 2007.

authorities recommend that this diagnosis should be based on identification of symptoms and signs suggestive of testosterone deficiency combined with presence of low testosterone levels measured by a reliable assay on two or more occasions.[135] Since testosterone levels vary with the time of day, being the highest in the morning (before 10 a.m.), they should be measured during this latter period to obtain the most meaningful values. If a single morning level is low or borderline low or does not fit with the clinical findings, the measurement should be repeated at least once or twice more before concluding that the levels are truly low. Consideration must be given to the overall context of man's age, coexistent diseases or obesity. Moreover, blood levels are dependent upon not only the testicular glands themselves, but also the pituitary gland (in the brain), which controls the ultimate output of testosterone. Because of such complexities, before embarking on treatment, individuals found to have ostensibly low blood testosterone levels are urged to seek a physician/specialist in endocrinology (glandular function), who will usually carefully analyze symptoms and perform more detailed study of blood testicular and pituitary hormones.

Testosterone replacement therapy should be avoided in men who still desire fertility. Aging males with a history of severe lower urinary tract obstruction, untreated sleep apnea, or prostate cancer should also avoid testosterone replacement therapy. Those with suspected prostate cancer, and/or elevated prostate-specific antigen (PSA) should probably not receive testosterone, or at least have a careful evaluation by a urologist before considering treatment.

The degree to which testosterone replacement is beneficial depends upon many factors. While some studies demonstrate

---

[135] Surampudi PN, Wang C , and Swerdloff R. *Hypogonadism in the aging male: Diagnosis, potential benefits, and risks of testosterone replacement therapy.* Int J Endocrinol. 2012; 2012: 625434.

increased muscle size and strength, and increased bone density, these results are inconsistent. Even if such changes occur, they could be non-specific in nature, similar to the steroid effects in athletes used to enhance performance.

The overall impact of testosterone replacement therapy on sexual satisfaction and erectile dysfunction (ED) is also unclear, varying among trials.[136] Long-term controlled studies are required to further evaluate these true effects.

The long-term benefits and risks of testosterone-replacement therapy will become clearer when the effects of testosterone are studied on all health-related outcomes over extended time. A large multicenter NIH (National Institutes of Health) supported double blind, placebo controlled study is ongoing, and this study should greatly enhance our knowledge about the efficacy and side effects of treatment.

Until more issues are resolved, I would caution men over the age of fifty against a headlong dash into such treatment, perhaps primarily because of the potential adverse effects on the prostate gland, especially in triggering or promoting the growth of cancer. Adverse cardiovascular outcomes, as well as other risks, remain largely unknown, but may also be looming over the horizon.

TELEVISION TESTIMONIALS—BRINGING FALLACIIES OF THOUGHT TO THE MASSES (SPREADING THE GOSPEL OF SELF-DESTRUCTION)

In May 2009, an attention-getting article titled "Live Your Best Life Ever!" appeared in *Newsweek*. The report was a microcosm of many of the myths I've already mentioned and deserves further discussion.

---

[136] Boloña ER, Uraga MV, Haddad RM, et al. Testosterone use in men with sexual dysfunction: a systematic review and meta-analysis of randomized placebo-controlled trials. *Mayo Clinic Proceedings*. 2007;82(1):20–28.

This article pointed out that in January 2009, Oprah Winfrey invited Suzanne Somers, a sixty-two-year-old actress, self-help author, and singer, to her popular television show to share her secrets to staying young, as well as other juicy tidbits aimed at achieving a better existence. So what were some of these secrets? Among others, they included Somers' rubbing a potent estrogen cream daily into the skin on her arm and smearing progesterone on her other arm two weeks a month. Her regimen included daily instillations of estrogens into her vagina with a syringe. The idea was to use unregulated bio-identical hormones to restore her hormone levels to what they were when she was in her thirties, thus fooling her body into thinking she's a younger woman. According to Somers, the hormones, which are synthesized from plants, are all natural and, unlike conventional hormones, virtually risk-free (which is patently false).

But that was only the beginning. Somers was taking sixty vitamins and other oral preparations every day. "I take about forty supplements in the morning," she told Oprah, "and then, before I go to bed, I try to remember…to start taking the last twenty." In her books, she says she also starts each day by giving herself injections of human growth hormone, vitamin B12, and vitamin B complex. Additionally, she wears "nanotechnology patches" to help her sleep, lose weight, and promote overall detoxification. If she drinks wine, she goes to her doctor to rejuvenate her liver with intravenous of vitamin C; if she's exposed to cigarette smoke, she has her blood cleaned with chelation therapy. Occupying the rest of her time is eating right, exercising, and relieving stress by standing on her head.

Somers makes astounding claims about the ability of hormones to treat almost anything that ails the female body. She believes they block disease and will double her life span. "I know I look like some kind of freak and fanatic," she said. "But I want to be there until I'm a-hundred-and-ten, and I'm going to do what I have to do to get there." Oprah, sitting next to Somers, dutifully defended her from attack by anyone in the audience. "Suzanne swears by bioidenticals and refuses to keep quiet. She'll take on anyone, including any doctor who questions her." This seemed to establish Oprah's scientific understanding (or lack thereof).

Somers further stated that mainstream doctors need to "get their facts straight." "The problem is that our medical schools do not teach this." She believes doctors, scientists and the media are all in the pocket of the pharmaceutical industry; "Billions are spent on marketing drugs, and these companies also support academic research." Free from these entanglements, Somers can see things clearly. "I have spent thousands of hours on this. I've written eighteen books on health. I know my stuff."

Although many dangerous myths have been spewed out repeatedly on this and other TV shows, this one could qualify for an Olympic scamathon in nonsense and chutzpah. If today's medical science were to adopt such a mentality, we would be back in the days of bloodletting and other such stupidity which had similar scientific credentials.

I raise this subject primarily to enumerate the flaws Somers demonstrated in her fallacious judgments, which are shared by far too many people.

1. Anecdotes never trump observational and rigorous scientific proof.

2. The intuitive logic that female hormones could produce significant long-term benefits has been largely debunked. These hormones, in the form of estrogen plus progestin, likely promote the development of breast cancer. Apparently Somers had already survived one bout of this type of cancer and is apparently oblivious to the additional risk she is assuming by using these hormones.

3 There is no evidence that favors bioidentical and natural products over those that are synthesized. On the

contrary, synthesized products are generally better analyzed and purified.

4 Daily multivitamins, as we have discussed, are useless—or even worse—unless one can't eat a decent diet.

5 Taking any treatment with the expectation of success is regularly followed by the placebo effect, which is enhanced if you are already a believer. I assume Somers did experience subjective gain following her various maneuvers.

6. Any perceived improvement following such a treatment would also be subject to the post hoc fallacy.

7. Chelation therapy is nonsense, as already noted.

8. Writing one or many books does not certify that one "knows her (or his) stuff."

Unfortunately, *Oprah* and shows like it provide a willing platform for far too many self-proclaimed experts willing to influence an uncritical public toward ill health and financial privation, if not danger. As *Newsweek* clarified "...the truth is, some of what Oprah promotes isn't good, and a lot of the advice her guests dispense on the show is just bad. The Suzanne Somers episode wasn't an oddball occurrence. This kind of thing happens again and again on *Oprah*. Some of the many experts who cross her stage offer interesting and useful information...Others gush nonsense. Oprah, who holds up her guests as prophets, can't seem to tell the difference. She has the power to summon the most learned authorities on any subject; and who would refuse her? Instead, all too often Oprah winds up putting herself and her trusting audience in the hands of celebrity authors and pop-science artists pitching wonder cures and miracle treatments that are questionable or flat-out wrong, and sometimes dangerous."

All I can add after this breathtaking betrayal of public trust is "Great job, *Newsweek*—you hit another home run!" But unfortunately I fear there are many more followers of Oprah and her ilk than *Newsweek* readers. Unfortunately, even though her program is gone, others continue to provide such misinformation and will likely do so for yet some time.

SECTION THREE: CONFUSION BETWEEN SCIENCE AND RELIGION

⟨⟩ *Chapter Nineteen* ⟨⟩

The Nature of Science

"The greatest discoveries of science have always been those that forced us to rethink our beliefs about the universe and our place in it."

Robert L. Park

For well over a century, many people of faith have been attacking scientists for certain theories that presumably deny the existence of God. This battle is perhaps most intense regarding Darwin's theory of evolution. To clear the confusion, we must first examine certain terms that play a central role in this conflict.

First, the word *science*, is derived from the Latin *scientia,* meaning knowledge. According to *Webster's New Collegiate Dictionary*, the definition of science is "knowledge attained through study or practice," or "knowledge covering general truths of the operation of general laws, esp. as obtained and tested through scientific method [and] concerned with the physical world." The scientific method uses observation and experimentation to describe and explain natural phenomena. Science also refers to the organized body of knowledge people have gained using that system. Less formally, the word science often describes any systematic field of study or knowledge gained from it. In all instances, the information gained is subject to confirmation, modification, and refutation by other investigators. It is universally agreed that scientific theories must be capable of being independently tested and verified by other scientists to become accepted by the scientific community.

But, analogous a sausage factory, scientific methodology is not clean and neat. As Carl Sagan[137] has aptly stated, "It is a supreme challenge for the popularizer of science to make clear the actual, tortuous history of its great discoveries and the misapprehensions and occasional stubborn refusal by its practitioners to change course. Many, perhaps most science textbooks for budding scientists tread lightly here. It is enormously easier to present in an appealing way the wisdom distilled from centuries of patient and collective integration of nature than to detail the messy distillation apparatus. The method of science, as stodgy and grumpy as it may seem, is far more important than the findings of science." Nowhere does this statement ring truer than in medical science.

BUILDING BLOCKS OF THE SCIENTIFIC METHOD: HYPOTHESIS, THEORY, AND LAW.

Hypothesis: This is an educated guess based on observation, a rational explanation of a single event or phenomenon based upon what is observed, but not been proved. Most hypotheses can be supported or refuted by experimentation or continued observation.

Theory: A scientific theory summarizes a hypothesis or group of hypotheses that have been supported with repeated testing and is valid as long as there is no evidence to dispute it, an explanation of a set of related observations or events based upon proven hypotheses and verified multiple times by detached groups of researchers. Having passed this rigorous testing, hypotheses become theory and, with rare exceptions, are generally accepted to be true.

---

[137] Sagan C. *The Demon-Haunted World*. Ballantine Books, New York, N.Y. 1997. p. 22.

Some scientific theories include evolution, relativity, the atomic theory, and the quantum theory. All of these theories are well documented and strongly supported beyond reasonable doubt. Virtually all scientists working in biological and related fields accept the validity of Darwin's theory of evolution, yet scientists continue to tinker with the component hypotheses of each theory in an attempt to make them more elegant and concise, or to make them more all-encompassing. Theories can be tweaked, but they are seldom, if ever, entirely rejected or replaced.

Scientific Law: This is a statement of fact meant to describe, in concise terms, an action or set of actions. It is generally accepted to be true and universal, and can sometimes be expressed in terms of a single mathematical equation. Scientific laws are similar to mathematical postulates. They don't really need any complex external proofs; they are accepted at face value because they have always been observed to be true.

Scientific laws must be simple, true, universal, and absolute. They represent the cornerstone of scientific discovery, because if a law ever did not apply, then all science based on that law would collapse. Scientific laws, or laws of nature, include the law of gravity, Newton's laws of motion, the laws of thermodynamics, Boyle's law of gases, the law of conservation of mass and energy, and Hook's law of elasticity.

In conclusion, I quote the words of Richard Feynman, world renowned physicist, who stated that "The principle of science is the following: The test of all knowledge is experiment. Experiment is the sole judge of scientific 'truth'. But what is the source of knowledge? Where do the laws that are to be tested come from? Experiment, itself, helps to produce these laws, in the sense that it gives us hints. But also needed is imagination to create from these hints the great generalizations —to guess at the wonderful, simple, but very strange patterns beneath them all, and then to experiment to check again whether we have made the right guess."

Feynman also observes, "…there is an expanding frontier of ignorance…things must be learned only to be unlearned again or, more likely, to be corrected." In general, the scientific method begins with a hypothesis, followed by a theory. This latter concept is sometimes confused with a scientific law.

From this explanation, one may conclude that science does not generate moral principles or prescribe moral behavior. Scientific techniques, however, can be applied to morality, primarily through the study of psychology, which constitutes one of the many branches of science. In this instance, investigators would not pass moral judgments—qualities of right or wrong—upon the information studied or the results obtained. For instance, psychological study might be applied to determine which background factors contribute most to a choice between honesty and criminal behavior, but science does not define morality per se.

THE LIMITS OF SCIENCE

How far can science go? We all encounter people who state that science doesn't have all the answers. But by stating such an obvious truth, they are often attempting to justify support of a mystical or religious belief. Critics often claim that if science cannot explain a given phenomenon, an alternative explanation is proved. Evolution is exquisitely illustrative of this, for creationists seek any perceived deficiencies in the theory of evolution to seize an alternative proof that divine intervention must have been involved. The same line of reasoning extends to all kinds of inexplicable phenomena that include paranormal phenomena such as extrasensory perception, extraterrestrial invaders, Marfa lights, and other bizarre ideas.

Science is the dynamic process of progressively furthering our knowledge in ever-expanding concentric rings of objective information. Because of the inexhaustible supply of questions about our universe, science, by definition, cannot ever have all the answers. If it did, science would cease to exist. The main principle is that when something happens that seems mysterious and unexplainable, it remains just that until objective scientific methods, when applicable, ultimately explain it or prove it to be a myth. Otherwise, in the absence of proof to the contrary, it remains a myth.

PSEUDOSCIENCE

Before leaving the topic of science, we must consider *pseudoscience*, which refers to a claim, belief, or practice presented as scientific, but which does not adhere to a valid scientific method, lacks supporting evidence or plausibility, cannot be reliably tested, or otherwise lacks scientific status. It is often characterized by the use of vague, exaggerated, or unprovable claims, a lack of openness to evaluation by other experts, and a general absence of systematic processes to rationally develop theories. While some religious doctrines at least partially fulfill this definition, it extends to all sorts of scientific misrepresentation. Sagan[138] presented an excellent list of criteria to detect such fraudulent methods, the most important of which are listed here.

1. Whenever possible, there must be independent confirmation of the facts.

2. Proponents of all points of view should engage in debate on the evidence.

3. Arguments from authority carry little weight. Authorities have made mistakes in the past, and they will do so in the future.

4. Consider alternative hypotheses. There is usually more than one explanation for a given phenomenon which must take into account and, whenever possible, be subjected to objective testing.

---

[138] Sagan C. *The Demon-Haunted World*. Ballantine Books, New York, N.Y., 1997, p. 210.

5. When possible, quantification should be applied. Numerical values allow better discrimination among competing hypotheses.

6. If there is a chain within an argument, every link in the chain must work, including the premise—not just most of them.

7. Always ask whether the hypothesis can be, at least in principle, falsified. Propositions that are untestable or unfalsifiable are worthless.

Pseudoscience includes some infomercials and interviews, but virtually all the claims made for alternative medicines and procedures.

The reliance on carefully designed and controlled experiments underlies the validity of all the statements above. We cannot learn much from contemplation alone. One is often tempted to be satisfied with the first possible explanation we can think of, but, in most instances, we can invent several. All cases require experimentation for their resolution.

❧ *Chapter Twenty* ❧

RELIGION AND ITS CONFLICT WITH SCIENCE

"This is my simple religion. There is no need for temples; no need for complicated philosophy. Our own brain, our own heart is our temple; the philosophy is kindness."

Dalai Lama

While not subject to a single or simple explanation, standard dictionaries define religion as "a set of beliefs concerning the cause, nature, and purpose of the universe, especially when considered as the creation of one or more supernatural beings usually involving devotional and ritual observances, and often containing a moral code governing the conduct of human affairs. In the case of western religions, this concept emanates from a single deity, i.e., God. In this latter instance, humans are believed to be created in the image of God; thus they are set apart from other living beings by possessing— among many other qualities—high intellect and the capacity for moral behavior."

Because the scientific concept of evolution, or the origin of humans, has been at loggerheads with some strict religious interpretations, we must explore this conflict in some detail. It pits the scientific view of evolution against common religious beliefs, often termed intelligent design or creation science.

CONTEMPORARY SCIENCE VERSUS CREATION SCIENCE

"Creationists make it sound as though a "theory" is something you dreamt up after being drunk all night."

Isaac Asimov

According to the scientific concept, evolution represents a long and usually gradual process whereby lower forms of life evolved through a process termed natural selection. What this means is that early life consisted of submicroscopic life-forms that manifested individual variations, probably mainly through a process of random mutations, or accidental variations of genetic makeup. While most of these changes resulted in inferior beings that did not survive, some resulted in modified physical features that were accidentally more favorable to survival. Individuals thus changed were more capable of survival and propagation to form a new class of beings better adapted to the existing environment.

How this living material began in the first place has been the subject of intense speculation, but in recent years plausible explanations have been elegantly reviewed by Dennet.[139] It likely began with prebiotic molecular material that, over a period of millions of years, developed the ability to replicate and pass through a period of natural selection, becoming progressively more complex, morphing eventually into DNA, which constitutes the genetic material of which all living cells are composed.

This process has gone on for millions of years and has accounted for vast forms of complex life, of which humans are one part. Scientific interrogation has determined that earth was formed approximately four billion years ago. In our present form, humans have inhabited this planet for approximately two million years. During this gradual and prolonged selection process, humans have developed relatively large and complex brains which have formed the substrate for higher intelligence. This latter feature is inextricably associated with the ability to form speech and language; moreover, the parallel development of fine manual dexterity allows for graphic displays and eventually written language.

---

[139]Dennet, DC, *Darwin's Dangerous Idea.* 1996, New York, N.Y. Simon and Schuster.

The ability to form language cannot be overemphasized, for it allows the brain to form and internalize arbitrary symbols that are used to represent external events and concepts. Such symbols (words and pictures) can be used to form an artificial internal world that comprises the process of thought (consciousness) and that allows us to project our reactions away from events in our immediate environment. This has enabled us to construct complex external structures, anticipate future events, learn from the past, and pass learning on to offspring and future generations. As a result of this function, humans now have the power to alter and decouple the evolutionary process from natural selection. For instance, medical science can preserve lives that would earlier have been nonviable, thus allowing these individuals to reproduce. The ultimate effects of these activities are unforeseeable, but they certainly are capable of contributing to worldwide problems such as overpopulation and impingement on the environment. Our activities also impact evolution indirectly through the production of global warming, which alters the global environment for many animal and plant species, ultimately creating unfavorable outcomes for many living beings.

Evolution can be replicated artificially over short periods by simply observing the response of many bacteria to various antibiotics. Shortly after these organisms are exposed to a given chemical agent, the vast majority are killed or rendered inactive, which provides the necessary improvement or cure of the disease in question. Because of biologic variability, however, a few of these bacteria have the capability to survive, then propagate, to form an entirely new colony that has the capability of warding off this given antibacterial agent. Within a matter of days or weeks, a given type of bacteria can evolve into an antibiotic resistant form. This provides us with not only a valuable learning experience but, from a practical standpoint, explains the need for avoiding the excessive and unnecessary use of antibiotics, and provides the impetus for searching for newer antibiotics.

In contrast, much religious dogma (at least fundamentalist) assumes that humans were placed upon this planet in their finished form approximately 6,000–8,000 years ago by an intelligent architect (God). Such a scheme is immutable and not subject to investigation or confirmation. The presupposed intelligent creator seems to be based on our understanding of intelligence as exemplified by the human model. Thus the concept that humans are created in the image of God, the cornerstone of much religious thought, appears to have been reversed—God has more likely been created by humans in their own image.

Does that mean that religions have become obsolete and are no longer relevant? No. All this information simply suggests most religions, to remain relevant, might best abandon this narrow, anthropomorphic, concept of God in favor of a broader, all-encompassing entity that rules the universe and probably even allows, and presides over, the process of evolution itself, providing us with the intellectual capacity to make observations and formulate theories about the process. As noted above, moral precepts will continue to emanate from religions and clearly fall outside of science. This does not mean, however, that one must be religious in order to be ethical, nor does it mean that being a scientist precludes a clear vision of what constitutes ethical behavior.

Most religious objections to scientific thought and methods probably stem from a profound respect and fear—as well as ignorance—of science. The element of respect probably accounts for the adoption of scientific names, such as creation science, which are used to gain a foothold in school science classes. Even the names of religious organizations themselves appear to be designed to convey a scientific aura, such as the Church of Scientology or Christian Science.

Early in the 20th century, there were active efforts by religious leaders to prevent the teaching of evolution in our public school systems, such as the Scopes trial, formally known as *The State of Tennessee v. John Thomas Scopes*. Because of the great interest this trial generated, then and now, I review it here briefly.

SCOPES TRIAL

In 1925, John Thomas Scopes, a biology teacher in Dayton, Tennessee, was arrested for violating an act of the state legislature which prohibited the teaching of evolution in schools. The American Civil Liberties Union took up the case, and America's most famous criminal lawyer, Clarence Darrow, defended Scopes pro bono.

Leading the prosecution was A. T. Stewart, the local district attorney, and William Jennings Bryan, the former presidential candidate. Bryan believed the literal interpretation of the Bible, and had been asked to take part in what became known as the Scopes Monkey Trial by the World Christian Fundamental Association.

The trial began in Dayton on July 11, 1925. Three schoolboys testified they'd been present when Scopes taught evolution in their school. When the judge, John T. Raulston, refused to allow scientists to testify on the validity of evolution, Clarence Darrow called William Jennings Bryan to the witness stand. Although Darrow successfully exposed the flaws in Bryan's arguments during cross-examination, Bryan was considered the nation's leading orator and was expected to shine during his summing up of the prosecution's case. To avoid this, Darrow decided against making a final summation, thereby robbing Bryan of this opportunity.

The jury found John Thomas Scopes guilty, and the judge fined him $100. Despite this, however, the verdict was overturned on a technicality and Scopes was never retried, providing a de facto victory for both Scopes and science. A successful Broadway play and movie, *Inherit the Wind* (1960), are based on the trial.

After these and other attempts to block the teaching of evolution were frustrated in the 20th century, the effort has now shifted toward attempts to introduce creation science into the curricula of standard science courses as an alternative explanation of evolution or, at minimum, to require teachers to issue a statement that evolution was merely a theory which remained unproven, thus suggesting religious interpretations might be valid. It is of interest to review briefly an example of this effort being tested in our federal court system.

KITZMILLER TRIAL

Tammy Kitzmiller, et al. v. Dover Area School District, et al. was the first direct challenge brought in the US federal courts against a public school district requiring presentation of intelligent design as an alternative explanation to evolution. The plaintiffs successfully argued that intelligent design is synonymous with creationism, both of which represent religious belief and violated the Establishment Clause of the First Amendment, i.e. . "Congress shall make no law respecting an establishment of religion"

Eleven parents of students in Dover, Pennsylvania, sued the Dover Area School District over a statement offering the option of intelligent design that the school board required to be read aloud in ninth-grade science classes when evolution was taught. The plaintiffs were represented by the American Civil Liberties Union, Americans United for Separation of Church and State, and Pepper Hamilton LLP. The National Center for Science Education acted as consultants for the plaintiffs. The defendants were represented by the Thomas More Law Center. The suit was tried from September 26, 2005 to November 4, 2005 before Judge John E. Jones III.

On December 20, 2005, Judge Jones issued his 139-page findings of fact and decision. He ruled that the Dover mandate was unconstitutional, and barred intelligent design from being taught in Pennsylvania's Middle District public school science classrooms. The judge's decision hinged primarily on the fact that intelligent design was not science, for it was not subject to objective analysis and confirmation, which made it a religious belief. The eight Dover school board members who voted for the intelligent design requirement were all defeated in the 2005 elections by challengers who opposed the teaching of intelligent design in science classes. The incumbent school board president said the board did not intend to appeal the ruling.

Perhaps the distinction here is that creationists, to counter the validity of science, must offer their own science to support their claims. Thus creationism itself would be open to falsification, which is clearly impossible.

I note with some irony that the plaintiffs were represented by the American Civil Liberties Union for, as noted above, Clarence Darrow was an early member of this organization.

✑ *Conclusions* ✎

D o the results of this litigation mean religion was defeated? No. But it does signal a serious setback for those who adhere to fundamentalist concepts of most religions. To function effectively in modern society, beliefs simply must be adapted to realities. Probably the best conciliatory statement in this regard was made by the late Pope John Paul II who, on October 27, 1996, stated in an address to the Pontifical Academy of Sciences in Rome, "Consideration of the method used in diverse orders of knowledge allows for the concordance of two points of view which seem irreconcilable. The sciences of observation describe and measure with ever greater precision the multiple manifestations of life…while theology extracts…the final meaning according to the Creator's designs."[140]

Was science the winner in this apparent conflict? No. Science is not in conflict with religion, since it seeks only to examine observable, palpable, and measurable factors. Just as science must continuously reevaluate its hypotheses and theories, discarding those proven false and forging onward to new unconquered territories, religion must modify its belief systems to accommodate to the ever enlarging body of knowledge gained through objective methods.

This controversy will continue for many years, especially regionally, but the outlook seems progressively bleak for creationists to succeed in public (and hopefully private) classrooms. My primary reason for this belief is derived from a recent Gallup poll which found that 40% of the US population believes God created man in essentially his present form within the last 10,000 years or so. Furthermore, Penn State political scientists

---

[140] Shermer M. *Why People Believe Weird Things*. St. Martin's Griffin, New York. 2002, p. 133.

Michael Berkman and Eric Plutzer reported in the Jan. 28, 2011 issue of *Science* that only 28% of 926 high school science teachers consistently follow National Research Council guidelines, which encourages them to present students with evidence of evolution. Surprisingly, 13% of these teachers "explicitly advocated creationism or intelligent design."

Given my background in the biologic and medical sciences, I feel qualified to add some additional comments. The underlying composition of building blocks of all life on this planet is strikingly similar. DNA is a complex submicroscopic structure that resides in the nuclei of cells, and contains the genetic instructions which direct the development and function of all known living beings, with the exception of some viruses. The main role of DNA molecules is the long-term storage of information, like a set of blueprints, or a recipe or a code, because it contains the instructions needed to construct other components of cells, such as proteins. The DNA segments that carry this genetic information are called genes, but other DNA sequences have structural purposes or are involved in regulating this genetic information. Thus DNA provides instructions to the cells regarding how they are to develop and what type of life they will form.

For instance, human DNA preordains its cells to develop into a complete human being. None of the components in this structure is unique, for every organ has a striking resemblance to a counterpart in the animal kingdom. Even our brains are not unique, for other species are endowed with very large and complex brains similar to those of humans. These include dolphins, elephants, great apes, and others. These observations detract further from the supposed and reverential uniqueness of humans within the animal kingdom.

᧪ *Epilogue* ᧫

With so many ways to arrive at erroneous conclusions, it's amazing we ever make correct judgments. In most instances, though, we are able to arrive at appropriate decisions which allow us to function effectively under differing circumstances. Very often, applying intuitive concepts, such as representativeness, can get us to the right destination when we are confronted by a new and unfamiliar situation. But, to avoid serious errors with potentially disastrous consequences, our methods of forming conclusions must always be analyzed and challenged. I hope that, through the examples presented in these pages, the reader will engage more actively in the recognition of and avoidance of common errors that lead to inappropriate personal decisions.

Although some prior knowledge of statistical principles is helpful in making judgments, one need not be a mathematician to appreciate the effect of large versus small numbers in inductive reasoning, the idea that most information is usually scattered in a bell-shaped configuration, and that chance factors are just what they are—having no real memory and no predilection to recur in a non-chance progression.

Science has progressed greatly over the past century, especially in biology and medicine. Through its methods we have forged a new path into disease prevention and treatment, which can shed light on the mechanism of apparent benefit provided by obviously worthless remedies. From an individual standpoint, however, s/he is usually primarily interested in obtaining relief from a symptom or disease. When apparent improvement follows a given intervention, one often attributes the result to the preceding act, which represents not only a potential post hoc error but also lack of understanding of the placebo effect, as well as the fact that most illnesses will improve or resolve with time in the absence of treatment. Faith healers and those providing "miracle" alternative medications can take advantage of these same principles, often to great financial gain. Even many of us in legitimate medical fields can intervene in some way—by pill or procedure—then may claim credit for the subsequent improvement or cure.

Although most of our treatments are supported by scientific rationale, we often have no way of separating physical from placebo effects. On occasion, most practitioners administer a treatment simply to obtain the placebo effect, accompanying the act with warm and encouraging words anticipating improvement. Since we all want good results when encountering such situations, a moral dilemma is created by the question of whether it is proper to inform a patient that s/he benefitted from a placebo effect, which may jeopardize the apparent improvement or relief. There is no answer to this ethical dilemma. Perhaps it was best summed up by a statement made many years ago by one of my colleagues and mentors, who said "It's OK to be a quack, as long as you know you're being a quack."

I conclude by reaffirming the title of this book; snake oil is alive and well. Similar to the case of atomic energy, however, our challenge is to learn how to harness the power of snake oil for good rather than for evil.

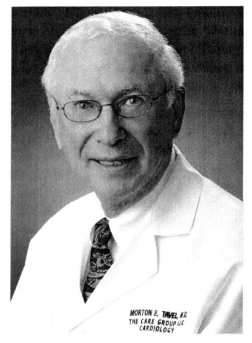

MORTON E. TAVEL, M.D.
THE CARE GROUP LLC
CARDIOLOGY

✐ *About the Author* ✎

D r. Tavel is a lifelong native of Indianapolis, having received both college and medical degrees at Indiana University. After completing his undergraduate studies, he graduated summa cum laude and was elected to the honorary scholastic society of Phi Beta Kappa. Upon completion of his medical training, he was elected to the Alpha Omega Alpha for scholastic achievement in this field. His post-graduate specialized training included stints in Philadelphia and Salt Lake City. After serving in the U.S. Army Medical Corps for two years in Germany, he returned to Indianapolis to complete has training and to begin medical practice.

Dr. Tavel is a physician specialist in internal medicine and cardiovascular diseases. In addition to managing patients for many years, he holds a teaching position (Clinical Professor) at Indiana University School of Medicine and regularly teaches medical students, house staff physicians, and other medical personnel. In addition, he has presented numerous speeches and lectures before national and international audiences that include peers as well as the general public. He is actively engaged in medical research and has authored over 100 research publications, editorials and book reviews that have appeared in peer-reviewed national medical journals. He is currently the director of the cardiac rehabilitation program at St. Vincent Hospital, Indianapolis, Indiana, and consulting cardiologist for the Care Group, Inc., a division of St. Vincent Hospital in Indianapolis.

Dr. Tavel has authored a book on cardiology that persisted through four editions over a period of approximately twenty years. This book was placed on the recommended list by the major U.S. internal medical organization (American College of Physicians) for inclusion in the personal libraries of all those practicing internal medicine. Dr. Tavel has also been a contributor to several other multi-authored textbooks. Having served on editorial boards of four major national medical journals, he has provided numerous critical reviews of manuscripts submitted to many journals for possible publication. He has also served as research director at a large metropolitan teaching hospital (Methodist Hospital), located in Indianapolis. His civic activities include, among others, having been past president of the local and state divisions of the American Heart Association, during which time he made numerous television and radio appearances on behalf of this organization. Many years ago, he was one of first to advocate restricting or eliminating smoking from public areas. Unfortunately, and much to his dismay, these efforts failed to reach fruition until the present era.

At present, Dr. Tavel is collaborating with a commercial enterprise in the development of a radically new stethoscope design that utilizes wireless computer and cell phone technology to record and transmit heart sounds and provide a platform for instruction of students.

All these activities do not prevent Dr. Tavel from engaging in an active personal life that includes travel with an educational focus, hiking, cycling, racquet sports, golf and fishing. Since he is a strong advocate of regular aerobic exercise, he has followed his own prescription in his endeavors for many years, activities that he hopes have provided motivation to both his patients as well as his trainees. He continues to reside in the Indianapolis area with his caring and supportive wife, Betty. And of course he would be remiss if he didn't mention that his collective family includes four children and eight grandchildren. Although in his book he probes in depth about the irrational formation of biases, he shamelessly boasts that his grandchildren are far above average in all respects.

Appendix

Bayes Formula (Modified)

Definition of terms:

Test sensitivity = The percentage of those having disease that test positive

or

number testing positive
number with disease

Test specificity = The percentage of those without disease that test negative

or

number testing negative
number without disease

Example Calculation

Method of calculating probability of disease, given a positive test result ("post-test probability," or P(D\+). This example assumes a prior (pre-test) probability of 10% and a test sensitivity of 90% and specificity of 90%.

$$P(D\backslash+) = \frac{\text{True Positives}}{\text{True Positives} + \text{False Positives}}$$

True positives = Proportion with Disease x Test Sensitivity
False positives = Proportion without Disease x False Positive Rate (1- specificity)

$$P(D\backslash+) = \text{post-test probability}$$

$$P(D\backslash+) = \frac{(0.9)x(0.1)}{(0.9 \times 0.1) + (0.1x.0.9)}$$

$$P(D\backslash+) = \frac{.09}{.18} = 0.5$$

Interpretation: Any individual with a positive test has a 50% (0.5) chance of having the disease.

Reversing the process in this example above, we analyze the chances that a given individual <u>without</u> the disease will have a negative test result, $P(D\backslash-)$

$$P(D\backslash-) = \frac{\text{True Negatives}}{\text{True Negatives + False Negatives}}$$

True Negatives = Proportion without disease x Test Specificity
False Negatives = Proportion with disease x (1- Test Sensitivity)

$$P(D\backslash-) = \frac{(0.9 \times 0.9)}{(0.9 \times 0.9) + (0.1 \times 0.1)}$$

$$P(D\backslash-) = \frac{.81}{.81 + .01} = 0.987$$

Interpretation: Any individual with a negative test has a 98.7% (.987) chance of being free of the disease.

CPSIA information can be obtained at www.ICGtesting.com
Printed in the USA
BVOW01s1639070814

361852BV00001B/115/P